ADOLESCENT MEDICINE:
STATE OF THE ART REVIEWS

E-Health

GUEST EDITORS

Alwyn T. Cohall, MD

Vaughn Rickert, PsyD

Owen Ryan, MPA, MIA

August 2007 • Volume 18 • Number 2

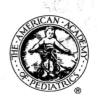

ADOLESCENT MEDICINE CLINICS:
STATE OF THE ART REVIEWS
August 2007
Editor: Diane E. Beausoleil
Marketing Manager: Linda Smessaert
Production Manager: Theresa Wiener, Shannan Martin

Volume 18, Number 2
ISSN 1934-4287
MA0393
SUB1006

Adolescent Medicine: State of the Art Reviews is published three times per year by the American Academy of Pediatrics, 141 Northwest Point Blvd, Elk Grove Village, IL 60007-1098. Periodicals postage paid at Arlington Heights, IL.

POSTMASTER: Send address changes to American Academy of Pediatrics, Department of Marketing and Publications, Attn: AM:STARs, 141 Northwest Point Blvd, Elk Grove Village, IL 60007-1098.

Subscriptions: Subscriptions to *Adolescent Medicine: State of the Art Reviews* (AM:STARs) are provided to members of the American Academy of Pediatrics' Section on Adolescent Health as part of annual section membership dues. All others, please contact the AAP Customer Service Center at 866/843-2271 (7:00 am–5:30 pm Central Time, Monday–Friday) for pricing and information.

Adolescent Medicine: State of the Art Reviews

Official Journal of the American Academy of Pediatrics
Section on Adolescent Health

EDITORS-IN-CHIEF

VICTOR C. STRASBURGER, MD, Professor of Pediatrics, Division of Adolescent Medicine, University of New Mexico, School of Medicine, Albuquerque, New Mexico

DONALD E. GREYDANUS, MD, Professor of Pediatrics, Michigan State University; and Pediatrics Program Director, Kalamazoo Center for Medical Studies, Kalamazoo, Michigan

GUEST EDITORS

ALWYN T. COHALL, MD, Director, Harlem Health Promotion Center and Project STAY, Mailman School of Public Health, Columbia University, New York, New York

VAUGHN RICKERT, PsyD, Professor, Heilbrunn Department of Population and Family Health, Mailman School of Public Health, Columbia University, New York, New York

OWEN RYAN, MPA, MIA, Graduate Research Assistant, Heilbrunn Department of Population and Family Health, Mailman School of Public Health, Columbia University, New York, New York

CONTRIBUTORS

RAQUEL ANDRÉS MARTÍNEZ, PhD, MSc, Department of Obstetrics and Gynecology, Columbia University Medical Center, New York, New York; and Centre for Research on Welfare Economics, University of Barcelona, Barcelona, Spain

DAVID BELL, MD, Departments of Pediatrics and Population and Family Health, Columbia University, New York, New York

WARREN K. BICKEL, PhD, HealthSim, LLC, New York, New York; and Center for Addiction Research, University of Arkansas for Medical Sciences, Little Rock, Arkansas

DINA L. G. BORZEKOWSKI, EdD, Department of Health, Behavior, and Society, Johns Hopkins Bloomberg School of Public Health, Baltimore, Maryland

PAULA M. CASTAÑO, MD, MPH, Department of Obstetrics and Gynecology, Columbia University Medical Center, New York, New York

ALWYN COHALL, MD, Harlem Health Promotion Center and Project STAY, Mailman School of Public Health, Columbia University, New York, New York

MARY-MARGARET H. DRISKELL, MPH, Pro-Change Behavior Systems, Inc, West Kingston, Rhode Island

DAVID FINKELHOR, PhD, Crimes Against Children Research Center, University of New Hampshire, Durham, New Hampshire

MICHAEL J. GRABINSKI, MCSD, HealthSim, LLC, New York, New York; and Red 5 Group, LLC, New York, New York

NICOLA J. GRAY, PhD, MRPharmS, Division for Social Research in Medicines and Health, School of Pharmacy, University of Nottingham, Nottingham, England

CARLY HUTCHINSON, BA, Harlem Health Promotion Center, Mailman School of Public Health, Columbia University, New York, New York

SHARIB KHAN, MBBS, MA, Department of Biomedical Informatics and Harlem Health Promotion Center, Mailman School of Public Health, Columbia University, New York, New York

JONATHAN D. KLEIN, MD, MPH, Division of Adolescent Medicine, University of Rochester, Rochester, New York

RITA KUKAFKA, DrPH, MA, Departments of Biomedical Informatics and Sociomedical Sciences and Harlem Health Promotion Center, Mailman School of Public Health, Columbia University, New York, New York

AIDAN MACFARLANE, FRCP, FRCPCH, FFPH, Oxford, United Kingdom

LISA A. MARSCH, PhD, Center for Drug Use and HIV Research, National Development and Research Institutes, New York, New York; and HealthSim, LLC, New York, New York

LEANNE M. MAURIELLO, PhD, Pro-Change Behavior Systems, Inc, West Kingston, Rhode Island

ANN MCPHERSON, CBE, MB, BS, FRCGP, DCH, Department of Public Health and Primary Care, University of Oxford, Headington, United Kingdom

KIMBERLY MITCHELL, PhD, Crimes Against Children Research Center, University of New Hampshire, Durham, New Hampshire

CAMERON D. NORMAN, PhD, Department of Public Health Sciences, University of Toronto, Toronto, Ontario, Canada

MONTSINE NSHOM, MPH, Harlem Health Promotion Center, Mailman School of Public Health, Columbia University, New York, New York

ANDREA NYE, MPH, Harlem Health Promotion Center, Mailman School of Public Health, Columbia University, New York, New York

DAVID M. N. PAPERNY, MD, FAAP, FSAM, Adolescent Clinic, Kaiser Permanente, and Department of Pediatrics, University of Hawaii School of Medicine, Honolulu, Hawaii

JANICE M. PROCHASKA, PhD, Pro-Change Behavior Systems, Inc, West Kingston, Rhode Island

VAUGHN RICKERT, PsyD, Heilbrunn Department of Population and Family Health, Mailman School of Public Health, Columbia University, New York, New York

OWEN RYAN, MPA, MIA, Heilbrunn Department of Population and Family Health, Mailman School of Public Health, Columbia University, New York, New York

KAREN J. SHERMAN, BA, Pro-Change Behavior Systems, Inc, West Kingston, Rhode Island

HARVEY A. SKINNER, PhD, CPsych, Faculty of Health, York University, Toronto, Ontario, Canada

ERIKA SUTTER, MPH, Division of Adolescent Medicine, University of Rochester, Rochester, New York

JANIS WOLAK, JD, Crimes Against Children Research Center, University of New Hampshire, Durham, New Hampshire

MICHELE L. YBARRA, MPH, PhD, Internet Solutions for Kids, Inc, Santa Ana, California

JEB WEISMAN, PhD, Departments of Sociomedical Sciences and Strategic Technologies, Mailman School of Public Health, Columbia University, New York, NY; and Center for Community Health Technology and Chief Information Office, Children's Health Fund, New York, NY

CONTENTS

> In this article, the development of 2 sophisticated health informa-
> tion and education initiatives geared at adolescents, children, and
> their families are described. These initiatives leverage advanced
> information technologies in concert with novel pedagogies, peer
> internship programs, and informal education methods to achieve
> the intended goals. The initiatives have been successful since their
> respective inceptions and will form exportable models for other
> organizations and institutions that seek to create similar opportu-
> nities and resources for adolescents.

> Electronic health records have been recognized as essential for
> improving clinical documentation, coordination, and manage-
> ment of health care in addition to lowering costs and improving
> patient safety. In recent years, there has been a significant im-
> petus for promoting the adoption of electronic health records, as
> evidenced by the numerous public and private initiatives across
> the United States. However, currently available electronic
> health records have not focused on the unique clinical, psycho-
> social, and health educational needs and requirements of the
> adolescent age group. In this chapter we discuss briefly the
> history, development, and adoption of electronic health records
> and provide examples of how electronic health records can be
> extended to focus on the needs of adolescents and those who
> care for them.

Office-Based Computerized Risk-Assessment and Health-Education Systems

David M. N. Paperny

Current computer technology and informational media formats can have dramatic effects on adolescent health. In this article, various advances and techniques used in adolescent health screening and assessment, as well as application of both common and advanced video and multimedia for health education and promotion, are reviewed. Future implications are discussed.

Secure E-mail Applications: Strengthening Connections Between Adolescents, Parents, and Health Providers

Alwyn Cohall, Carly Hutchinson, Andrea Nye

Although e-mail has become a popular means of communication among consumers, particularly youth, available evidence suggests that current use of this modality to facilitate communication between consumers and their health providers is relatively modest. Historically, structural and legal issues have provided substantial impediments; however, new developments in providing secure and protected mechanisms for transmitting and delivering e-mail messages may pave the way to enhance use and improve communication.

PART 2: TECHNOLOGY AND RESEARCH

Internet Surveys With Adolescents: Promising Methods and Methodologic Challenges

Erika Sutter, Jonathan D. Klein

The use of Web-based surveys and methods has grown substantially in recent years. Internet surveys have the potential to produce data rapidly and efficiently, provide access to hard-to-reach populations, and reduce response biases. Although some methodologic questions require further exploration, Web-based survey methods can accurately represent many adolescent and young-adult populations and will be an increasingly relevant part of how we learn about the attitudes and behaviors of youth in our society. This article reviews current literature and some of the strengths and limitations of Web-based survey research with adolescent and young-adult populations.

There are 2 ways to think about emerging technology and adolescent health research. First, one can try to understand the relationship between technology and adolescent health. This line examines whether time spent using emerging technologies or being exposed to messages and applications are associated with poorer or better health. The second way looks at how technology is and can be used through delivering interventions, data collection, or analyses. This article examines both ways of thinking. Given the limited (albeit growing) number of published studies, we use a case-study approach to illustrate relationships and methods. After discussing the purpose and findings, we highlight a study's strengths and weaknesses, not to praise or disparage a researcher's work but to critique the research. We conclude by describing common concerns in adolescent research suggesting ways to advance the field of emerging technologies and adolescent health research.

We review current knowledge about adolescent Internet-mediated victimization, including Internet-initiated sex crimes in which offenders use the Internet to meet victims, unwanted online sexual solicitations, Internet harassment, and unwanted and wanted exposure to online pornography. Internet-initiated sex crimes have received considerable publicity, but the media stories have contributed to stereotypes that do not accurately portray adolescent Internet experience. Adults' concerns are valid but need to be supported with information that illuminates the real safety issues and targets the specific population of youth impacted.

PART 3: TECHNOLOGY AND BEHAVIORAL INTERVENTIONS

This article provides an overview of several interactive, computer-based substance abuse–prevention and –treatment interventions that we have developed for adolescents, including an interactive substance abuse–prevention multimedia program for middle school–aged youth and a customizable program focused on prevention of HIV, hepatitis, and sexually transmitted infections among youth in substance abuse treatment. The content in these programs is grounded in a scientific understanding of the types of skills and information that are critical to effective prevention. The programs also use several evidence-based informational technologies that have been shown to be critical in effectively training key skills and information. Our evaluations to date have underscored the effectiveness of these programs in producing desired health-behavior change. Applying information technologies to the delivery of science-based interventions may allow for unique opportunities to provide widespread dissemination of cost-effective interventions with consistency and in a manner that is engaging and acceptable to youth.

Since 1995, TeenNet Research (www.teennet.ca) has been a leader in developing strategies for involving youth and adults in co-creating e-health–promotion Web sites and behavior-change programs. In this article we review TeenNet's experience and lessons learned from more than a decade of action research with youth, with an emphasis on the guiding frameworks for participatory action research and Web-site creation and evaluation. The models are applied to the Smoking Zine (www.smokingzine.org), a 5-stage Web-assisted tobacco intervention, which is profiled with regards to its development, evaluation, and dissemination, including results from a school-based randomized, controlled trial. The prospects for using information technology to engage youth in health promotion are discussed in relation to TeenNet's past work and future interests in new Web 2.0 technologies.

In this article, the development of the concept and measurement of "off-line" health literacy is charted, recent development and interest in adolescent off-line health literacy is explored, and how the Internet could be useful in assessing and improving adolescents' online and off-line health literacy skills is considered. The important issue of content filters will also be considered as it relates to adolescents' ability to retrieve online health information about sensitive issues.

The use of interactive technologies to promote health behaviors is a rapidly expanding field. Yet, the integration of these technologies in the development of physical activity and nutrition interventions for adolescents is in its infancy. *Health in Motion*, a multimedia obesity-prevention program for adolescents, is described as a case example of a Web-based interactive program for promoting physical activity and fruit and vegetable consumption among high school students. Lessons gathered from existing programs are summarized and used to offer future direction for advancing the development of adolescent interventions in this field.

Sexually active adolescents are at risk for unintended pregnancy. Teen pregnancies can be prevented by consistent use of birth control, such as oral contraceptives. However, many teens forget their daily doses and eventually stop using oral contraceptives altogether. Teen pregnancies are more likely to be medically complicated and can adversely impact the teen, her child, and their community. Cell-phone use is becoming widespread, and teen cell-phone users frequently use text messaging. We describe a study in which we use cell-phone text-messaging technology in a novel way: we provide daily oral contraceptive dosing reminders and educational messages and evaluate oral contraceptive continuation at 6 months. We will use the information we obtain to develop specific, practice-based interventions to improve reproductive health programs and policies.

The Internet is an exciting resource for providing immediately available, evidence-based, health information for young people in an age-appropriate form on a 24 hours/day, 7 days/week basis. www.teenagehealthfreak.org is a United Kingdom–based Web site designed to take advantage of this. The content of the site, which is the leading teenage health Web site on a Google search, contains both the diary of a hypochondriac 15-year-old boy and a virtual doctor's surgery. It also allows for young people to e-mail health-related questions and receive relevant answers from a health expert. Analysis of the content of these e-mails indicates the unmet health needs and concerns of young people. Future developments of the site include linking the site www.youthhealthtalk.org, a Web site that contains videotaped interviews with young people who have a variety other health concerns.

Youth development programs have the potential to positively impact psychosocial growth and maturation in young adults. Several youth development programs are capitalizing on youths' natural gravitation toward technology as well. Research has shown that youth view technology and technologic literacy as positive and empowering, and that youth who master technology have increased self-esteem and better socioeconomic prospects than their counterparts. Technology-centered youth development programs offer a unique opportunity to engage youth, thereby extending their social networks, enhancing their access to information, building their self-esteem, and improving their self-efficacy. This article provides an overview of the intersection between youth development and technology and illustrates the ways technology can be used as a cutting-edge tool for youth development.

Preface

E-Health

Technological advancement and its integration into everyday life profoundly affect how we entertain, learn, and communicate. For example, instead of purchasing a CD of a favorite band or vocalist (or a vinyl record for those of us who are really old), we can log onto a computer and use a secure connection to purchase and download a song or album from the Internet onto our MP3 player or iPod without ever having to leave the comfort of our office or living room. But beyond entertainment, technological advancements have the potential to impact learning and communication about health. For example, "[m]ore than any other communication medium or health-related technology, the Internet has the greatest potential to promote health and prevent disease for individuals and communities throughout the world."[1] Many adults are turning early and often to the Internet for information, support, and guidance about health care matters. Adolescents are similarly predisposed and likely more adept at obtaining information from this source.

> These amazing, mysterious, and rapidly emergent young people who both charm and confound us might very soon be our partners, employees, or even managers, but they'll definitely become—if they aren't already—our prospects and customers. Do we have any real clue about how they will interact with technology, and it with them, in the coming few years? Are we prepared to think and behave in the new ways that such, uh, different customers will require?[2]

Although this quote refers to the intersection of the business community with adolescents, it is relevant to their health as well. As health providers, public health practitioners, educators, and advocates for young people, it is important that we understand and appreciate how adolescents think about and use all the technology available to them. We, as professionals, must develop strategies to maximize the potential of technology to play significant roles in enhancing adolescent health and well-being.

We have divided this issue into 3 sections. The first section, "Technology in Clinical Care," examines the development and implementation of electronic systems designed to improve clinical interactions between health care providers and adolescents in a variety of care settings such as hospitals, mobile vans, clinics, and private offices. The second section, "Technology and Research," addresses how innovations in technology can be integrated into adolescent health research. We have tried to offer illustrations of how technology can be used to gather information from adolescents as well as more sophisticated methodologic approaches to examine the effect that technology has on the health and well-being of adolescents. The final section, "Technology and Behavioral Interventions," uses a case-based format to identify and highlight cutting-edge examples of how computer and Web-based interactive programs have been designed to support innovative adolescent health promotion activities. In addition, the section explores opportunities for using technology to attract and retain young people in youth development initiatives.

As co-editors, we gratefully acknowledge the support of Drs Strasburger and Greydanus, who helped to shape and conceptualize this edition of *AM:STARs*, and Diane Beusoleil and her staff for their editorial assistance. In addition, we thank all of our contributing authors who worked diligently and creatively to prepare an excellent array of thoughtful articles that provide a useful foundation that can be applied to youth around the globe to enhance and improve their health and well-being.

Alwyn T. Cohall, MD
Harlem Health Promotion Center and Project STAY
Mailman School of Public Health at Columbia University
New York, New York

Vaughn Rickert, PsyD
Heilbrunn Department of Population and Family Health
Mailman School of Public Health at Columbia University
New York, New York

Owen Ryan, MPA, MIA
Heilbrunn Department of Population and Family Health
Mailman School of Public Health at Columbia University
New York, New York

REFERENCES

1. Bernhardt JM. Health education and the digital divide: building bridges and filling chasms. *Health Educ Res*. 2000;15:527–531
2. Evans B. Teens' inscrutable adventures. *InformationWeek*. January 7, 2002. Available at www.informationweek.com/story/showArticle.jhtml?articleID=6500767. Accessed August 1, 2007

Adolesc Med 18 (2007) 231–245

Novel Implementations of Information Technology in Support of Adolescent Health Knowledge Acquisition: 2 Cases

Jeb Weisman, PhD*

Department of Sociomedical Sciences and National Center for Disaster Preparedness, Mailman School of Public Health, Columbia University, 722 West 168th Street, New York, NY 10032, USA

Center for Community Health Technology and Chief Information Office, Children's Health Fund, 215 West 125th Street, Suite 301, New York, NY 10027, USA

The initiatives described herein combined technology, education models, and human services in a tertiary inpatient pediatric hospital and a school-based ambulatory primary care setting. Targeted research work was performed that encompassed the development of eclectic end-user technical systems that support a variety of learning styles and curriculum models. In concert, these elements formed sophisticated networks of teaching, knowledge acquisition, and behavior-modification opportunities. These opportunities were leveraged to teach children, adolescents, and their families about arrays of ideas and topics while exposing them to previously unknown or misunderstood aspects of their world and life choices. Especially emphasized areas included life skills, artificially delimited categories of information referenced as personal health, community health, and public health knowledge and strategies, and an introduction to global ideas critical to adolescents' lives in an increasingly interconnected world community.[1–4] I was the chief architect of both of these initiatives and managed the operations of the hospital-based program for 3 years after it opened.

CASE STUDY: 2 CASE ENVIRONMENTS

The first case environment was designed as part of a children's hospital that opened in the fall of 2001, and the second was designed as part of an interdisciplinary school-based health facility that opened in 2006. The cases served different target populations in terms of health status (inpatient versus ambulatory), physical environments (children's hospital versus school-based clinic), and age groups (~0–21 vs ~12–18 years). The underlying design, education, and

*Corresponding author.

E-mail address: jweisman@chfund.org or jw2199@columbia.edu (J. Weisman).

technology philosophies were similar. The school-based facility was designed by using lessons acquired from the hospital project.

Initiative 1: Children's Hospital at Montefiore, 2001

In the late 1990s, the Board of Trustees and management of Montefiore Medical Center determined that demographic and market changes within their service area (the Bronx and southern Westchester County, NY) exposed a significant need for a children's hospital to provide emergency, specialty, and inpatient care for the 0- to ~21-year-old local population (2000 US census estimates reported ~1 330 000 known residents: 337 315 0- to 15-year-olds and 201 560 16- to 24-year-olds[5]). Plans for the Children's Hospital at Montefiore (CHAM) coincided with the national technology "boom." Within months, the Internet became integral to popular culture and, in turn, informed design decisions related to CHAM. Montefiore Medical Center's extensive investment in health information technologies matured to a point at which broad distribution and mandated use were strategically, practically, and economically viable. Intentions for CHAM to embrace health information technologies from its inception were formalized in terms of its mission and planning process.

In 1998, additional mandates were added by the medical center's leadership that, among other things, were meant to engage the patient population in activities that are not typically identified with hospitals. Two opportunities emerged. The first was to provide a higher level of medical and health integration between the primary care sites and the hospital to embrace a family-centered care philosophy.[6,7] The belief was that children and their families are active partners in the health care process; the health of a child is measured not only in medical terms but also from perspectives of psychosocial, economic, intellectual, and life opportunity and action. The second opportunity was that the facility might embody a broader sense of health and life opportunity than was traditionally embedded in tertiary care models. A novel vision to engage many sectors of the patient population in nontraditional activities was articulated.[8] One aspect of this philosophy came to be called the Carl Sagan Discovery Program (CSDP).

The CSDP was intended to provide a breadth of experience through which patients and their families were introduced to ideas and information that encompassed general health and a generically identified "world of ideas" not otherwise accessible in their daily lives. The hospital and the CSDP engaged the physical architecture[9] of the building, organization of the floors and operational processes, and a program of informal education, information technology, and peer mentorship.

At the opening of CHAM and continuing forward, the CSDP used features from patients' inner city multicultural environments to draw connections to their lives, interests, and opportunities not previously experienced, internalized, or critiqued. To do this, we developed a series of learning goals and objectives based on various state and national education criteria and National Aeronautics and Space Administration educational objectives. We then designed an information system that was capable of supporting these objectives and a human resources model to support both the education plan and the technical system. Three years of field research and testing were performed to ensure that screen designs accommodated not only patients and families ranging in age from 3 years through adulthood but also variations in languages.† Indeed, the system is capable of delivering materials in a virtually limitless number of languages, depending only on the availability of source material in the relevant language or dialect. The information system's underlying relational database management system allows for long-term storage and retrieval of user records to accommodate the entirety of a patient's relationship with the hospital.

Physically and operationally, hospital floors are organized by function in the case of the critical care unit (CCU), day hospital, and outpatient subspecialty clinics. Inpatient floors are segmented by general age (children, adolescents, and infants). Social work staff, allied health professionals, and mandated New York City teachers are located throughout the floors.

Technology

A 42-inch flat-panel display is located on the wall opposite each patient's bed. Next to the bed is a SmartCard reader (Fig 1) and a wireless keyboard. This equipment enables access to a television, a video-on-demand system that contains movies and educational content, and an interactive portal into a virtual environment called the Explorer Network (EN). Access is available throughout the hospital, including the lobby. Regardless of where the SmartCard is used, the user's profile customizes and personalizes the experience so that even if the card is removed, the system will start at precisely where the last activity ended; this supports continuity of experience and ownership.

As patients use the EN, the software tracks and learns their interests. The system then suggests alternative interactive paths of entertainment and inquiry. These suggestions often seem unrelated to the way the patient has been using the system. In fact, the system uses Bayesian algorithms[10,11] to make nonlinear suggestions, approximations of interest, and statistical best guesses as part of the process of exposing the user to a greater array of information and entertainment opportunities. Over time, the knowledge base about a patient's interests and activities grows. If a patient returns some years later, the EN will suggest resources that reflect not only known interests but also those that reflect advancement in age since the previous encounter. If a patient becomes the parent of a child who enters the hospital, the EN will remember the former patient and also connect the child to that parent.

---

†For example, as a written language, Spanish occupies ~25% more space than its English equivalent.

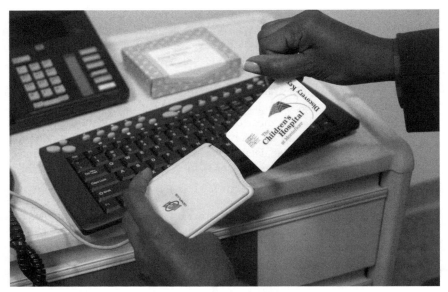

Fig 1. SmartCard reader and EN SmartCard. (Photo courtesy of Jeb Weisman, PhD.)

Interaction

All of the CSDP technology, content, and educational processes are supported by the explainers. The Explainers Program is an ongoing, extended-term, compensated internship program. It is an integral part of the CSDP that competitively recruits high school– and college-aged students from the surrounding community. The program incorporates a rigorous preparation program that trains the selected adolescents in the theory and practical fundamentals of teaching, working in a hospital environment, patient psychology, culture, and social factors that influence their experience and the experiences of their hospitalized peers. They are also instructed in the necessary legal and policy issues, privacy and confidentiality measures, and coping skills for working with acutely ill and dying patients. At the conclusion of the training process, explainers complete a practicum and are true docents; they can triage technology issues, describe in detail the features of every aspect of the hospital, act as teachers and mentors to the patients and the patients' families, and partner in curriculum, content, and technology development. The CSDP professional staff, in turn, oversees and supports all aspects of the technical, educational, and docent work.

The interactive environment uses a set of customized open-source technologies (eg, OpenACS [based on the Ars Digita Community System]) running though a switched 1-gigabyte ethernet hybrid fiber and copper network.

Process

After a patient's admission to the hospital, the CSDP is electronically notified, and a SmartCard is customized for the new patient. Returning patients may bring their card with them or request a replacement card. At a time convenient to the patient, an explainer visits to deliver the card. He or she then begins the patient-education process. The visit begins with technical instruction—how to use the card to activate the system, search for content, interact with the various communication technologies, and manage the ancillary systems such as television and video-on-demand. In fact, a very different instructional process is taking place.

Our early and continuing research has shown that virtually every adolescent who entered the hospital was computer literate enough to figure out the mechanics of the system in short order. However, we also discovered that, along with technical literacy, there is an extremely rigid, concrete understanding of information technology–based resources. Adolescents will tend to be very familiar with the technical process of achieving a specific goal, such as visiting a Web site or finding a song. In general, however, they will not link separate ideas and concepts together to use the systems to develop novel responses to information needs. In addition, their capacity to perform online research is extremely limited by a poor understanding of research practices in general and how to evaluate the quality and accuracy of what they discover. Combined with a culturally ascribed status as "victim,"[12,13] often associated with patient status and the general disorientation and discomfort resulting from the condition that brought them to the hospital, this tendency toward a familiar concreteness undermines an extraordinary opportunity for new experiences and understanding. It is the task of the explainer to jump-start the process to effectively exploit this captive opportunity.

At the time CHAM opened, the average length of stay for a patient was 3.2 days and remains in this range. During that period, the patient will sleep on the order of a total of at least 24 hours, may be recovering from anesthesia, and may be in pain or in some other health-related state or activity including formal patient education and training that requires attentiveness. Effectively, the CSDP has ~6 hours during the 3.2-day period to make a lasting impression on the patient (for returning patients, a somewhat longer period of interaction is possible). As a result, the goals evolved less to provide in-depth education about specific topics; rather, the goals are to expand individuals' understandings of information-finding techniques, to significantly broaden their opportunities to see and interact with the world outside of their typical experience, and to offset the alienation[14] and victim status associated with pediatric patients' experiences during hospitalization.

The information technology that was developed and is visually and technically engaging becomes a "hook" to attract and direct the patients along an intended path. The explainer, beginning the technical orientation, inserts the SmartCard into the bedside reader. The system opens up on the bed's display, greeting the patient by name and quietly organizing content by the patient's developmental age group (Fig 2). The explainer may ask the patient what kind of music he or she likes and then demonstrate how to find and play that music and learn about an artist. Next, the explainer connects the music to the actual experience of singing and then to the physiologic processes that singing requires. This, in turn, may allow a parallel to some sort of physical exertion or activity such as mountain climbing or hiking. From there, the feeling of breathlessness is developed into a sense of personal experience that is similar to the feeling of an asthma attack, which forms a link to the event that brought the patient to the hospital. The explainer creates indirect, informal, abstract-to-concrete connections that embody complex concepts and concrete experience in accessible ways. This forms the basis of a critical Web of information, understanding, and personal experience and establishes a rapport between the explainer, patient, and often the family as well (all of whom may have SmartCards). To support future activities, the EN is designed to accommodate point-to-point and multipoint videoconferencing by using technologies such as iVisit[15,16] and Skype.[17,18]

Having entered into the education and conceptual indoctrination process, the patient receives a series of visits throughout his or her stay. Explainers track their visits and maintain an ongoing information log to ensure that as shifts and staffing change, there is continuity of experience for the patient or family member. Notable is the fact that these visits are virtually the only contacts the patient will have during that time that are not formally connected to the medical reason for the inpatient status. This is often reflected in patient and family comments to staff and in the poststay consumer evaluation process.

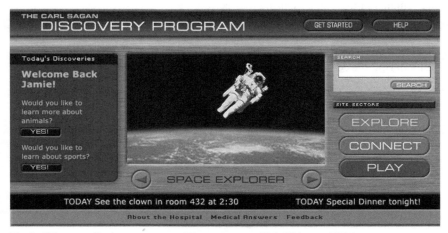

Fig 2. EN personalized access screen. (Photo courtesy of Jeb Weisman, PhD.)

Clinical Anecdotes

During the fist 3 years of operations, many successful anecdotes were catalogued. In 1 case, a 14-year-old Hispanic girl was hospitalized for a 5-day stay. Her 2 adolescent female siblings were often seen in attendance during school hours. The siblings and patient were reported to be successful students who enjoyed school. On questioning, the sisters explained that their mother felt they learned more at the hospital from the explainers and the EN than they did in school. The underlying reasons may as likely be linked to parental concerns that the patient would be well served if her siblings were present; nonetheless, the environment was perceived to be adolescent friendly and of arguably substantive educational value.

In another case, the CSDP and explainers were contacted about delivering the EN technology to an ethnically Middle Eastern 16-year-old boy who was awaiting a transplant on extended stay in the CCU. The patient was depressed and had virtually stopped eating and interacting with the hospital staff, which affected his opportunities for the transplant. During the CHAM planning phase, the CSDP and EN were not included in the CCU. The CSDP team designed a mobile version of the EN technology for the patient. For the medical staff, it was believed that the technology alone would offer a solution for the depression. However, once the explainers delivered the system, their training helped to develop a rapport with the patient. They approached nutrition and nursing staff to design a diet that was suggestive of his culture's cuisine, engaged him socially each day, and redirected his attention from the newspaper's obituary section to the EN. As a result, within 24 hours his outlook changed substantially, and he received the transplant successfully and later became an explainer himself. Many patients have subsequently applied to become explainers, and virtually all of the explainers have changed their post–high school plans to include college.

Today the CSDP and its human and technology resources are inextricably linked to education and to the health-delivery process at CHAM. Notable is the use of technology to engage patients and their families in a larger process of learning, health, and socialization.

Initiative 2: Harlem Children's Health Project, 2006

In 2006, the Harlem Children's Health Project (HCHP) opened in New York City as an integrated part of the Promise Academy charter school.‡ The HCHP provides health services for the community's school-aged population in areas of primary, mental health, and dental care as well as social work services, subspe-

---

‡According to the National Center for education statistics, a charter school is defined as "a publicly funded school that, in accordance with an enabling state statute, has been granted a charter exempting it from selected state or local rules and regulations. A charter school may be newly created, or it may previously have been a public or private school; it is typically governed by a group or organization (eg, a group of educators, a corporation, or a university) under a contract or charter with the state."

cialty referral services, and health education.

Incorporated into the HCHP is the Health Promotion Leaning Lab (HPLL). The HPLL was designed to target unique education opportunities for the Promise Academy's adolescent student populations, especially in areas of health and science. Peer and informal science-education styles of learning have long been discussed as effective means of teaching.[19–23] The HPLL's goals are to teach the students and their families about personal, community, and public health and to coordinate health and allied science teaching activities with the work of the HCHP health educator and the Promise Academy's teachers.

To meet its mission, the HPLL uses an integrated program of information technologies, a well-defined pedagogy and curriculum, and informal science-educational models. Similar to the CSDP, it leverages an explainers internship program to manage the facilities, participate in content development, and create teaching resources and lesson plans that are age and culture relevant. The technology used in the laboratory involves a variety of systems: several cabinet-mounted 42-inch flat-panel displays (inside the entryway, waiting area, and workspace) and personal computer workstations (Fig 3) that provide productivity applications, Internet access, and video-conferencing capabilities. They are also fashioned with screen-saver software that contributes to global research on, among other things, AIDS, tuberculosis, and cancer. In the center of the waiting area is a projection system mounted in the ceiling that projects down onto a floor screen that is ~7 square feet.

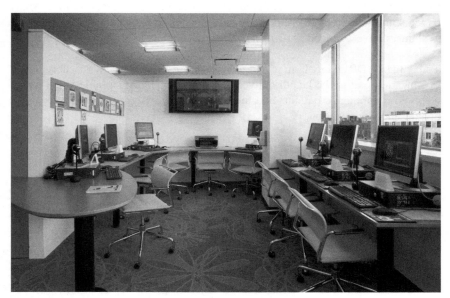

Fig 3. HPLL laboratory workstations. (Photo courtesy of Jeb Weisman, PhD.)

The entry hall displays act not only as broadcasters of information but also as 2 stations in a video game we call *The Daily Beat*. The video game uses heart monitors adapted from exercise equipment. Players each hold a sensor set and try to move particles that look like blood cells from his or her display to the opponent's display. To speed the process, players must learn to relax, reducing their heart rates to increase the particle flow through virtual space. They must develop physiologic self-awareness and develop techniques for controlling their heart rates. Once they find successful body-mind control strategies, adolescents have proven particularly adept at internalizing their solutions to win the game.

The display in the waiting area uses its capture camera to read objects, people, color, contrast, and movement in near proximity. The changing information is fed into a system called Swarm. Swarm continuously updates an on-screen abstract "painting" of those objects using vibrant colors. The process of repainting uses algorithms that are based on the movement of schooling fish and flocks of birds. Images can also be printed as souvenirs.

The display over the laboratory area incorporates an audio/video-capture device and Internet links to external sensor data. The screen presents an animated street seen of Harlem called Window on Harlem. It includes local landmarks including the nearby elevated railway, the historic Apollo Theater, and the Promise Academy. The visual style is reminiscent of a collage made of art that is based on the Harlem Renaissance tradition. The capture device reads sound near the display and translates it into increased animated traffic on screen (buses, pedestrians, cars). The more sound, the busier the Harlem scene. At the same time, the capture device transmits changes in color and light in the environment to alter the background of the scene as it scrolls by. The colorful clothing of those in front of the display will similarly change the image's background color. Externally acquired data change the scene as a real-time response to the external world, as well. As the sun actually sets, street lights in the displayed simulacrum come on, the train station lights up, and the trains themselves show internal lighting in the passenger areas. As the sun rises, the light goes off. If it rains or snows outside, the on-screen window on Harlem similarly mirrors these meteorologic changes and the pedestrians open umbrellas for protection.

The floor projection system is called the Sea of Ideas. Projected from above, any image file can be displayed. These images are created by the students and explainers. Motion sensors read movement in the area of the floor projection. As people move through the projected image, it responds by fragmenting, with pieces of the image flying away and then reintegrating to reform the whole.

All of the displays and installations are integrated and can be accessed from separate locations. In this way, teachers and students can centralize and manage the teaching/learning process and share their creations and work. Similarly, the workstations have the ability to video-conference with anyone in the world as long as the participant at the other end has access to an inexpensive video camera and Internet connection.

The HPLL is accessed by students in a variety of ways, none of which are mutually exclusive. First, some students participate as they come to the HCHP for health care. Their interaction with the system is inherently limited, because they may be feeling ill or may require some level of isolation to reduce the transmission of disease. In this case, the Swarm, Window on Harlem, and Sea of Ideas systems are ideal. They allow patients to remain relatively passive yet integrate their presence into the interactive output. In so doing, the system engages the adolescent and sets an impression that remains long after the encounter. The experience also destabilizes traditional perceptions of school-based and other primary care clinics, hopefully establishing the foundation for a broader-based set of assumptions and understandings.

Second, students visit and participate in the HPLL as part of organized classroom learning excursions. The manageability and flexibility of the technology allows the staff educator, explainers, and classroom teacher to organize a lesson with clear objectives and skills but using informal science-education methods. Activities that would be difficult within a traditional classroom or inaccessible in an inner-city environment can be created, simulated, or extended in the HPLL. Not only does this add value to the classroom curriculum, but it also connects the abstractions of classroom health and science education to the practical realities of health care operations.

Students access the laboratory a third way as part of independent study activities. School faculty and students visit to develop their understandings of the HPLL's technical and human resources, which establishes the facility as an independent study project destination.

Finally, students access the HPLL on their own during their free time. In these cases, they participate in informal, guided learning opportunities. To draw a parallel with current marketing techniques, they become a means to virally transmit[24,25] ideas about the HPLL, explainers, and opportunities to others.

In all cases, student participation is limited to prearranged class schedules or nonprogrammed time. As the adolescent students' comfort and familiarity with the HPLL grow, they begin to bring family members to the HCHP, which reinforces the community-resource nature of the facility and helps to strengthen the process of redefining the nature of health care. It also legitimizes their time spent at the facility, which reinforces their likelihood of taking full advantage of the content and techniques available. The HCHP, through its HPLL, seeks to establish student and family understandings of health as concerns and practices that extend beyond episodic care or traditional learning modalities. The HPLL creates an opportunity to engage the people it serves in issues of personal and public health, many of which are unseen or formally inaccessible through school and in economically disadvantaged environments. In effect, it supports consumers of both health services and public health knowledge.

The HPLL has been operating for ~9 months. During this period, referred to as phase I, curriculum development and refinements have been taking place. After 12 months, phase II will begin with a full evaluation and the initiation of new technologies and projects.

OBSERVATIONS ABOUT THESE INITIATIVES

In both the CSDP and HPLL projects, technology has been tightly bound to a model of teaching that emphasizes informal science education, practice-based internships, and student activities. This model stands in some contrast to other common models. In the first instance there is what we may call the computer-laboratory model. In this case, the idea of information technology and the content it could enable is reified—concretized as the physical computer object. In the second instance, a structured science-education model is used in which testing is emphasized over integration with creative internalized processing. In the former instance, the technology itself becomes the focus of activities, defining all that may or may not be accomplished, confusing the potential with a physical tool. The enabling facility tends to be described in terms of its technology (eg, "computer laboratory"), activities center on the computers, or other technologies themselves, and the educators are sometimes less sophisticated in their appreciation and understanding of the technical systems than the students; the computer dictates what may or may not be learned and by whom. In the latter instance, a clearly defined framework and set of curricular objectives drives the education process. These objectives are the primary focus. Secondary learning and processing of tangential/nonlinear ideas are minimized or avoided altogether to accommodate pressures of time and measurable objective-centered performance, which results in a focus on a set of testable answers without a concomitant development of necessary critical-thinking/analysis-application skills.

Certainly much criticism has been aimed at the computer-laboratory model.[26–30] As well, there are substantial governmentally driven bases for the existence of the rigidly bounded objectives-driven approach.[31,32] The HPLL/CSDP approaches provide an integrated alternative to these approaches. Used alone or as part of a collaborative informal education process, these broad-based coalitions of technology, people, and pedagogy can spur interest and support creative exploration and understanding of sophisticated health-related topics. Indeed, as part of the curriculum process, the HPLL uses the question "can this activity or objective stand on its own if information technology is unavailable?" to measure how they are conceptualizing an element for inquiry in the program.

MEASUREMENT

These initiatives have provided a unique opportunity to measure success. To move beyond merely anecdotal information, 2 evaluation models are being tested for use during HPLL's phase II. The first derives from the established field of informal science-education research. Instruments and techniques exist to measure and describe the effectiveness of museums and similar facilities.[33–35] The second model draws from the field of actor network theory, popularized by a variety of researchers including Latour,[36] Callon,[37] and Law and Hassard.[38] This is a substantially more involved process in which the actors, agencies, and processes are mapped dynamically to clarify the constellation of relationships that are the basis for the subject under examination. Success is determined by watching the actors' relative significance through proximity and dominance change in the network map as methods and tools are brought into or removed (in this case, from the process of education). This evaluative and visually descriptive method helps participants understand how the dynamics of their program work and uncovers forces that may go unnoticed in purely quantitative measurement systems. This system of evaluation is expected to help to describe the novel nature of the HPLL and may be applied to the CSDP.

ADDITIONAL CONSIDERATIONS AND THE FUTURE

Another strategy for the use of information technology in educational and behavior-modification projects is described through captology.[39–41] Although the fundamental theme, computers as persuasive technology, is consistent with the overall goals of the CSDP and the HPLL, it is not a guiding precept at this time. To date, the focus at the CSDP and the HPLL has been on creating integrated pedagogies through which to build and enforce nonlinear thinking, theoretical knowledge applied to personal life circumstances, abstract associations, and a general understanding of the relevance of various health and scientific concepts to adolescent life. In particular, using information technologies, including computers, without building an educational program dependent on them for initial success has been a central intent. It may be that during future phases of these programs' operations they will undertake focused captologic projects. This will require an increased emphasis on the aspects of information technology as an autonomous aspect of these programs, semi-independently seeking to change user behaviors.

CONCLUSIONS

It is my experience that although information technologies present an opportunity to instill sophisticated public health information, all too often the novelty and excitement of the tools that are built become ends unto themselves. In this role, they obscure the original purpose for which they were created and derail the educational promise of the pedagogy. It is vital, then, that the linkage between educational intent and technology be created from a systematic perspective, acknowledging that both sets of needs are part of a dynamic system of material, process, and agency. Decoupling technology, pedagogy, and curriculum should leave a vibrant program of education that can stand on its own. This is a litmus test for a sustainable program that endures beyond its material elements. This requires engaged, sophisticated (knowledgeable) educators, an appreciation for the capabilities and limits of information technologies when integrated into educational programs, a willingness to test novel learning modalities, and the technical and human willingness to adapt to what is learned and changing exigencies.

It is helpful to remember that the subjects of our work, adolescent men and women, are undergoing an intense period of physiologic, psychological, and environment change, adjustment, integration, and adaptation. We must expect our own models and institutions to accommodate these changes and to use our resources to optimize our responses to maximize our positive impacts. Our technologies and the systems in which they are embedded reflect our capacity to adapt to the needs of our users, not the other way around. That responsibility is ours.

REFERENCES

1. Larson RW. Globalization, societal change, and new technologies: what they mean for the future of adolescence. *J Res Adolesc*. 2002;12:1–30
2. Blum R, Nelson-Mmari K. The health of young people in a global context. *J Adolesc Health*. 2004;35:402–418
3. Jensen LA. Coming of age in a multicultural world: globalization and adolescent cultural identity formation. *Appl Dev Sci*. 2003;7:189–196
4. Arnett JJ. The psychology of globalization. *Am Psychol*. 2003;57:774–783
5. US Census Bureau. United States Census 2000. Available at: www.census.gov/main/www/cen2000.html. Accessed January 30, 2007
6. American Academy of Pediatrics. Family-centered care publications. Available at: www.medicalhomeinfo.org/publications/family.html. Accessed January 30, 2007
7. Lawlor MC, Mattingly CF. The complexities embedded in family-centered care. *Am J Occup Ther*. 1998;52:259–267
8. LaBarre P. Strategic innovation: the Children's Hospital at Montefiore. *Fast Company*. 2002; 58:64. Available at: www.fastcompany.com/magazine/58/innovation.html. Accessed May 9, 2007
9. Weisman J. Performing hospitals from the ground up. *Perform Res*. 2004;9:66–70
10. Bernardo JM, Smith AFM. *Bayesian Theory*. Chichester, United Kingdom: Wiley; 2001
11. Heckerman D, Geiger D, Chickering DM. Learning Bayesian networks: the combination of knowledge and statistical data. *Mach Learn*. 1995;20:197–243
12. Macnab AJ, Thiessen P, McLeod E, Hinton D. Parent assessment of family-centered care practices in a children's hospital. *Child Health Care*. 2000;29:113–128
13. Chaudhury H, Mahmood A, Valente M. *The Use of Single Patient Rooms vs. Multiple Occupancy Rooms in Acute Care Environments: A Review and Analysis of the Literature*. British Columbia, CA: Simon Fraser University; 2003
14. Velazquez JM. Alienation. *Am J Nurs*. 1969;69:301–304
15. Pagram J, Fetherston T, Rabbitt E. Learning together: using technology and authentic learning experiences to enhance the learning of distance education students. In: *Proceedings of the*

Australian Indigenous Education Conference. Fremantle, Australia: Edith Cowan University; 2000

16. iVisit LLC. iVisit. Available at: www.ivisit.com. Accessed January 30, 2007
17. Karahali KG, Viégas FB. Social visualization: exploring text, audio, and video interaction. In: *Proceedings of the Conference on Human Factors in Computing Systems.* New York, NY: ACM Press; 2006
18. Skype Limited. Available at: www.skype.com. Accessed January 30, 2007
19. Milburn K. A critical review of peer education with young people with special reference to sexual health. *Health Educ Res.* 1995;10:407–420
20. Woods ER, Samples CL, Melchiono MW, et al. Boston HAPPENS Program: a model of health care for HIV-positive, homeless, and at-risk youth. Human immunodeficiency Virus (HIV) Adolescent Provider and Peer Education Network for Services. *J Adolesc Health.* 1998;23(2 suppl):37–48
21. Turner G, Shepherd J. A method in search of a theory: peer education and health promotion. *Health Educ Res.* 1999;14:235–247
22. Wellington J. Formal and informal learning in science: the role of the interactive science centres. *Physics Educ.* 1990;25:247–252
23. Fadigan KA, Hammrich PL. A longitudinal study of the educational and career trajectories of female participants of an urban informal science education program. *J Res Sci Teach.* 2004;41: 835–860
24. Phelps JE, Lewis R, Mobilio L, Perry D, Raman N. Viral marketing or electronic word-of-mouth advertising: examining consumer responses and motivations to pass along email. *J Advert Res.* 2004;44:333–348
25. Welker CB. The paradigm of viral communication. *Inf Serv Use.* 2002;22:3–8
26. Wilson BC. A study of learning environments associated with computer courses: can we teach them better? *J Comput Sci Coll.* 2004;20:267–273
27. Orlikowski WJ. The duality of technology: rethinking the concept of technology in organizations. *Organ Sci.* 1992;3:398–427
28. Orlikowski WJ, Robey D. Information technology and the structuring of organizations. *Inf Syst Res.* 1991;2:143–169
29. Warner J. What should we understand by information technology (and some hints at other issues)? *Aslib Proc.* 2000;52:350–370
30. Wild M. Technology refusal: rationalising the failure of student and beginning teachers to use computers. *Br J Educ Technol.* 1996;27:134
31. US Department of Education. No child left behind. Available at: www.ed.gov/nclb/landing.jhtml. Accessed January 30, 2007
32. Texas Education Agency, Student Assessment Division. The Texas Assessment of Knowledge and Skills . Available at: www.tea.state.tx.us/student.assessment/index.html. Accessed January 30, 2007
33. Online Evaluation Resource Library. Available at: http://oerl.sri.com/home.html. Accessed January 30, 2007
34. Sadler TD. Informal reasoning regarding socioscientific issues: a critical review of research. *J Res Sci Teach.* 2004;41:513–536
35. Rennie LJ, Johnston DJ. The nature of learning and its implications for research on learning from museums. *Sci Educ.* 2004;88(S1):S4–S16
36. Latour B. *Reassembling the Social: An Introduction to Actor-Network-Theory.* New York, NY: Oxford University Press; 2005
37. Callon M. The role of hybrid communities and socio-technical arrangements in the participatory design. *J Cent Inf Stud.* 2004;5:3–10
38. Law J, Hassard J, eds. *Actor Network Theory and After.* Malden, MA: Blackwell Publishing, Inc; 2006
39. Fogg BJ. *Persuasive Technology: Using Computers to Change What We Think and Do.* Burlington, MA: Morgan Kaufmann; 2002

40. Berdichevsky D, Neuenschwander E. Toward an ethics of persuasive technology. *Commun ACM.* 1999;42:51–58

41. Chan AS. Health captology: application of persuasive technologies to health care. *Stud Health Technol Inform.* 2004;106:83–91

Adolesc Med 18 (2007) 246–255

Extending Electronic Health Records to Improve Adolescent Health

Rita Kukafka, DrPH, MA[a,b,c,*],
Sharib A. Khan, MBBS, MA[a,c], David Bell, MD[d,e],
Jeb Weisman, PhD[b,f], Alwyn Cohall, MD[b,c,d,e]

Departments of [a]Biomedical Informatics, [d]Pediatrics, [e]Population and Family Health, and [b]Sociomedical Sciences, Columbia University, 622 VC5 West 168th Street, New York, NY 10032, USA

[c]Harlem Health Promotion Center, Mailman School of Public Health, Columbia University, 215 West 125th Street, New York, NY 10027, USA

[f]Children's Health Fund, 215 West 125th Street, Suite 301, New York, NY 10027, USA

The medical record has traditionally served as the definitive document that describes the clinical record of a patient and has a central role in care planning, monitoring, coordination, and communication. The earliest mention of keeping such records goes back many centuries, but the modern-day record has its origins in the Flexner report on medical education, which described its functions and contents.[1] The advent of computers in the 1940s and 1950s paved the way for the transformation of the medical record, from paper to electronic, beginning with the classic report by Ledley and Lusted, who described the potential use of computers in medicine.[2] The development of the Technicon Medical Information System (TMIS) set the stage for developing the precursors of today's sophisticated clinical information systems and electronic medical record (EMR) systems.[3] The Computer Stored Ambulatory Record (COSTAR), one of the first EMRs, was implemented at the Massachusetts General Hospital in 1968.[4] Lawrence Weed, who pioneered the concept of a problem-oriented medical record, developed the PROMIS system to support this paradigm of documentation.[4] These developments were followed by other significant system-building efforts at several academic medical centers: the Health Evaluation Through Logical Processing (HELP) system at LDS Hospital in Salt Lake City, Utah, and the Regenstrief Medical Record System at the Regenstrief Medical Center in Indianapolis, Indiana. Vista, one of the most successful electronic health record (EHR) systems, is still used by Veterans Affairs more than 2 decades after it was first developed.

*Corresponding author.
E-mail address: rita.kukafka@dbmi.columbia.edu (R. Kukafka).

Over the past 3 to 4 decades, EHR systems have evolved from being mere data repositories to include sophisticated documentation, decision support, and other features such as lifelong record keeping instead of episodic reporting. Several landmark reports, particularly *The Computer-Based Patient Record*[5] and *Crossing the Quality Chasm*,[6] coupled with rising costs of health care have led to a growing adoption and mainstreaming of EMR/EHRs.

WHAT IS AN EHR?

There is no standard or accepted definition of what constitutes an EHR, but it is important to emphasize that an EHR is not just an electronic representation of the paper record. Briefly, it can be described as a software system that supports broad categories of function:

1. electronic documentation of clinical notes, laboratory, and radiology information and clinical order entry;
2. integrated view of clinical data (EHRs can list and summarize clinical information such as medications prescribed or laboratory results and can also provide clinical parameter trends analysis, such as changes in a patient's cholesterol or hemoglobin A1c levels over time);
3. decision-support capabilities in the form of drug-drug interaction alerts, preventive care alerts or clinical documentation, and note-taking reminders (some systems provide even more sophisticated evidence-based guidelines to supplement clinical decision-making and patient management);
4. workflow and communication tools such as patient scheduling, calendaring, and referrals management to support interoffice communication;
5. reporting tools to examine aggregate patient data, which then can be used in quality assurance or service-delivery monitoring;
6. provision for representation and coding of clinical information (most systems today include standard terminologies such as the *International Classification of Diseases, Ninth Revision* (ICD-9) to code medical events, and these codes can be tied to other systems [such as the billing system to generate bills]);
7. security features such as authorization mechanisms, access controls, and audit trails to provide adequate safeguards to protect the confidentiality of information;
8. facilitation of interoperability with other systems by using recognized standards for data representation and exchange;
9. patient education (includes a repository of health education materials that can be printed out for the patient as well as Web-based links to knowledge resources); and
10. patient self-management tools (EHRs are increasingly being extended to include a personal health record component that allows patients to

interact with their medical record and enable them to maintain daily blood pressure or diet logs).

In addition to this basic description of what an EHR can do, there are 2 well-known EHR specifications that address the important and needed functionality required in such systems. One such specification is the EHR functional model developed by Health Level Seven, a globally recognized health care information technology standards organization.[7] The other requirements checklist was developed by the Certification Commission for Health Information Technology,[8] a nonprofit organization entrusted by the Department of Health and Human Services to develop the criteria to evaluate the functions supported by an EHR system. Today, there are a plethora of software vendors that provide a wide spectrum of systems under the EHR category. In general, most systems can be classified as serving outpatient or inpatient settings. They can also be classified as serving the needs of general clinical care or those of specific specialties such as pediatrics, surgery, or oncology.

BENEFITS OF USING AN EHR

One of the main benefits of using an EHR derives from the move from a paper-based documentation system to an electronic one. Although paper as a medium for information storage has several advantages (such as ease of use and familiarity), it has several disadvantages (such as difficulty in enforcing structured or standard documentation practices) that can be complicated even further by a lack of legible information. Paper does not facilitate data-integrity checks (being able to automatically detect incorrect values for a parameter) or enable decision support or the ability to mine a large number of records for clinical outcomes rapidly. Data recorded on paper usually reside in one place and cannot be readily transmitted or copied, which makes care coordination difficult. The EHR overcomes all of these limitations, because it stores information digitally, which makes the records amenable to different views, complex data mining, or easy transferability to facilitate care coordination.

Besides providing the advantage of an electronic medium for information storage, retrieval, and dissemination, EHRs have been documented to improve patient safety, decrease costs, promote the use of clinical guidelines, enhance communications among care providers, and promote public health activities.[9-11] Health care cost savings through EHRs are realized through a reduction of repetitive tests, suggestions for alternative procedures or medications, and, in the long run, by promoting better management of chronic conditions. A cost-analysis study conducted in an ambulatory primary care setting reported a range of savings from $2300 per provider to a net benefit of $330 900 per provider over a 5-year time period.[9] Likewise, patient safety can be improved through decision-support tools. For example, a systematic review showed that EHRs combined with electronic decision-support tools can reduce the frequency of adverse drug interactions.[10]

The increase in accessibility of information brought about by the EHR helps increase productivity. In an early study of EHR systems, the University of Wisconsin Hospital and Clinics reported that its system reduced nurse intake time for an initial outpatient visit from 35 to 20 minutes and reduced intake time for return visits from 35 to 15 minutes.[11] Recent initiatives are beginning to use the EHR as a tool to aid public health surveillance (evidenced by pilot projects initiated under the Primary Care Information Project at the New York City Department of Health and Mental Hygiene) and improve recruitment for clinical trials.[12]

ADOPTION AND IMPLEMENTATION CHALLENGES

Despite the potential benefits, EHR adoption can be described, at best, as slow. In the last few years, efforts have intensified to make this technology, classified as "essential" by the Institute of Medicine, more broadly available. Currently, only 20% of hospitals and 17% of provider clinics use EHRs.[13] A recent study of 526 pediatricians revealed that only 21% used EHRs in their practice. Those that did tended to be larger, networked practice settings.[14]

The primary barrier to adoption and implementation has been financial. The initial fixed costs, including hardware, software, training, and other setup, can be hundreds of thousands of dollars for even a small practice,[15] which makes EHR systems prohibitively expensive for these providers. In addition, providers bear the cost of technology without receiving any of the realized cost-savings benefits from the insurance providers.

There is also a perceived or realized loss in productivity that results from changes in the workflow after the introduction of a new system. Some studies have found adverse effects of EHR implementation on productivity, whereas others have reported on how deficiencies in system design (eg, complex data-entry forms in a computerized order entry system) can induce physician error.[16]

Market instability among vendors and in the technology sector is in itself a major barrier to adoption. Many health care executives are hesitant to invest in EHR systems, because they are waiting for better technology and market stability in the volatile health care information sector.[17]

Pediatric providers are concerned about the lack of available decision support such as prompts for delivery of appropriate immunizations.[14] However, in those model systems that have a complete array of features, providers who use EHRs have been shown to conduct more preventive health screening (eg, lead exposure, vision and hearing) and have higher rates of counseling parents about important health issues than their peers who use conventional paper records.[18] In an effort to make electronic systems more useful to pediatric practices, the American Academy of Pediatrics Council on Clinical Information Technology has joined with others to call for standardization of the features of EHRs and a certification of their functions.[19,20]

CURRENT EHR-ADOPTION INITIATIVES

In the last few years, there have been several notable initiatives aimed at promoting the adoption of EHRs. President Bush publicly committed to encouraging the use of EHRs universally and established the Office of the National Coordinator for Health Information Technology in 2005 to promote this effort. New York City initiated a project to provide low-cost EHR systems to providers serving in community clinics under the Primary Care Information Project,[21] and the Massachusetts eHealth Collaborative (www.maehc.org) began a demonstration project to implement interoperable medical records systems throughout the state. Several other organizations like the Markle Foundation (www.markle.org) and the California Health Care Foundation (www.chcf.org) are promoting and funding projects related to EHR adoption.

EXTENDING EHRs TO INCLUDE ADOLESCENT NEEDS

There are currently more than a hundred EHR systems available commercially or otherwise. However, most systems lack the necessary data models (which are needed to define and store information in a system) to incorporate special clinical issues related to adolescent health. Similarly, there is a paucity of research detailing the functional requirements of an EHR to support adolescent privacy needs. At most, research and vendor product development have focused on the pediatric age group. Several commercial systems include special modules in their EHRs that cater to the specific needs of the pediatric population such as maintaining a growth chart or immunization record.

The following sections discuss why it is important to propose extensions to the current EHRs and describe extensions that could potentially improve adolescent health.

Why Adolescents?

Population-based surveys have found that adolescents engage in a variety of health-compromising behaviors such as a sedentary lifestyle, unhealthy dieting, unprotected sexual intercourse, substance use, and reckless driving.[22] Risky behavior in these areas contributes to the leading causes of adolescent morbidity and mortality and sets a pattern for future health problems during adulthood.

To assist clinicians in caring for youth, a variety of protocols, tools, and approaches have been developed; however, the extent to which these guidelines have been implemented in clinical practice varies. Studies have shown that adolescents are reticent about discussing health issues with a clinician, but most would welcome supportive guidance from their provider.[23] These practitioners, however, are missing opportunities to deliver preventive care in part because of inexperience and lack of training in evaluating adolescents.[24,25] A well-designed EHR system could prove useful in filling this void.

Extending the EHR Clinical Data Model

Using the framework outlined previously as a general guide, we have attempted to describe how an adolescent EHR (AEHR) could be designed to specifically meet the needs of adolescents and their providers. Where necessary, categories are combined.

1. Electronic documentation: The AEHR could use forms derived from the *Guidelines for Adolescent Preventive Services*[26] to create a standardized intake form, providing clinicians with a comprehensive biopsychosocial profile of the adolescent. Such a profile could highlight areas of strength and underscore areas in need of focused attention.
2. Decision-support capabilities: In addition to providing prompts to remind providers about administering standard immunizations on a timely basis, the system could be structured to alert practitioners to opportunities for discussing new products with adolescents and parents, such as the human papillomavirus vaccine. In addition, structured fields could be incorporated to remind the clinician to inquire about key risk-taking behaviors (such as sexual activity) at each visit. In addition, for those adolescent girls found to be sexually active, the AEHR could automatically schedule a timetable for reminding the provider to conduct pelvic examinations for pap smears and sexually transmitted infection screens. Such a system would assist many practices in becoming more compliant with Health Plan Employer Data and Information Set (HEDIS) measures. Given the significant overlap between psychosocial, behavioral, and biological issues during adolescence, the system would be equipped to encourage clinicians to consider a range of possibilities when an adolescent presents for evaluation of headaches or abdominal pain.
3. Reporting tools: Continuing with the example listed above, with the AEHR the provider would be able to run periodic reports to determine the number of girls aged 11 to 18 years in the practice who may be eligible for the human papillomavirus vaccine. Such a report may help in ordering supplies and sending out announcements. In addition, with respect to sexually transmitted infection screening and pap smears, internal reports could be generated to determine rates of service provision and focused attempts made at correction before external auditing.
4. Patient education/self-management: This feature would allow clinicians to augment their one-on-one patient education and counseling time with tailored fact sheets, which could provide detailed health information on contraceptive options, sexual health, etc. Providers can steer youth toward credible Web resources to obtain more information. For those young women choosing the birth control pill as a method of choice, the system could (via secure e-mail) send periodic encouragement and reminders to enhance adherence, as well as receive feedback from the adolescent (such as compliance logs), which the provider could review and store in the electronic record.

5. Workflow and communication tools/interoperability/integration of clinical data: In addition to standard scheduling features, the interoperable AEHR could facilitate exchange of information between primary care providers and subspecialists. Current paper charts are clumsy, cluttered, and confusing, which makes timely and coordinated communication difficult. Primary care providers may not know the latest changes in insulin regimen or hemoglobin A1c levels of their diabetic patients. Endocrinologists may not know that the primary care provider initiated Depo-Provera because the patient became sexually active. Having an organized and legible record wherein all medications and laboratory values are listed along with provider notes, queries, and concerns may improve overall patient care and management. Similarly, an interoperable AEHR would facilitate transfer of information between primary care providers who are responsible for the patient at different times of the year (eg, the camp or college health provider and the adolescent's primary care provider). Those adolescents for whom transfer of information needs to occur between institutions (eg, juvenile justice/detention or chronic care/rehabilitation) or for determination of benefits (Supplemental Security Income/disability) would also be well served in this manner.

6. Clinical encounter coding: To improve revenue generation, the AEHR would have the *International Classification of Diseases, Ninth Revision* and *Current Procedural Terminology* codes that are most relevant to the provider who cares for adolescent patients and would also have the appropriate evaluation and management codes to improve billing and revenue generation.

7. Security features: The AEHR needs to offer increased protection of sensitive and confidential health information regarding reproductive health issues, substance use, and mental health concerns. In many states, adolescents have the right to obtain confidential services without parental notification and may limit the release of certain elements of their medical record to parents and other authorities.[27] To ensure that confidential information is not compromised, AEHR developers might choose to include pop-up reminders regarding limited-access information and audit systems that track access to patient files.

A MODEL EXAMPLE

The following EHR model has been operational for several years.

The Children's Health Fund (CHF) is a unique organization that provides and advocates for better health care for children both internationally and in the United States. For the latter, CHF delivers care to children and families through a system of both stationary and mobile health clinics. They provide a "medical home" to youth who are struggling to survive in the most difficult of circumstances in areas as varied as the south Bronx, New York, and rural West Virginia. Since 1990, the program has logged >1 240 000 visits.

To better evaluate clients and coordinate delivery of care, the CHF developed an EMR called EHRIS (Electronic Health Record Information System) in 1999. The system is expected to capture all the information considered critical to traditional medical records along with broader historical, educational, and psychosocial information that comprises more expansive notions of health (see Fig 1 for an example). As the clinician checks boxes that apply to the patient's condition, the system writes the record in intelligible English. For example, "Amanda is a 26-year-old female. She is the reporter. Her primary language is English, etc." All of the computed information is maintained in a "container" that supports the Health Information Portability and Accountability Act (HIPAA).

Among the data captured are demographics, appointment and procedure scheduling, procedures, procedure results, standard indicators for charting and the resultant graphical charts (eg, growth charts, BMI), immunizations, insurance/billing data and interactions, subspecialty referral management and associated scheduling activities, medical and health encounter (visit) data, prescription and prescription writing, laboratory orders and their results, health education, alternative therapies, and other relevant patient information. Links are made between patients who are members of the same family, their parents, and/or equivalent caregivers. Additional modules include an online virtual classroom that integrates with the health record and a system that provides detailed logistic handling

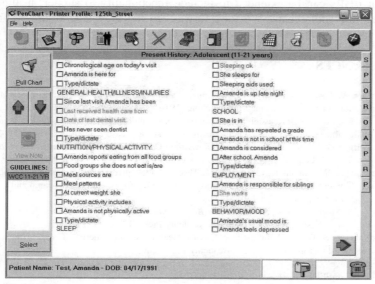

Fig 1. Model EHR screenshot.

of the subspecialty referrals, associated appointments, and implicit complex transportation and communications processes required to ensure compliance. All data are fully accessible for reporting, analysis, and interpretation. The collected data are intended, in various formats, for 4 audiences operating in a specific clinical context:

1. health care providers and their staff using a traditional medical-record metaphor;
2. health care program administrators, primarily through standardized grid and exportable reports to support operational functions including productivity, trends, etc;
3. researchers, advocates, and policy analysts, primarily through standardized grid and exportable reports with all personal identifiers stripped out; and
4. health care consumers and their immediate families, in a format to be determined but supportive of portable records data and emergency preparedness.

The main focus of clinical content development has been with pediatric and adolescent patients. Several key expectations regarding accessibility and confidentiality have been established by program coordinators to ensure that system development adheres closely to patient and provider needs.

CONCLUSIONS

EHRs are essential to delivering quality health care and are being increasingly adopted across hospitals and provider clinics. However, most current EHRs are not built to support the health issues pertaining to adolescents, which are a very important demographic group. We have outlined several ways in which the current EHRs can be extended to include functionality to support health care delivery for adolescents. We look forward to the very near future when the AEHR becomes standard practice in providing services for youth.

REFERENCES

1. Flexner A. *Medical Education in the United States and Canada*. New York, NY: Carnegie Foundation for the Advancement of Teaching; 1910
2. Ledley RS, Lusted LB. Reasoning foundations of medical diagnosis: symbolic logic, probability, and value theory aid our understanding of how physicians reason. *Science*. 1959;130:9–21
3. Shortliffe EH, Cimino JJ. *Biomedical Informatics: Computer Applications in Health Care and Biomedicine*. 3rd ed. New York, NY: Springer; 2006
4. Fitzmaurice JM, Adams K, Eisenberg JM. Three decades of research on computer applications in health care: medical informatics support at the Agency for Healthcare Research and Quality. *J Am Med Inform Assoc*. 2002;9:144–160
5. Dick RS, Steen EB, eds. *The Computer-Based Patient Record: An Essential Technology for Health Care*. Washington, DC: National Academy Press; 1991
6. Institute of Medicine, Committee on Quality Health Care in America. *Crossing the Quality Chasm*. Washington, DC: National Academy Press; 2001
7. Health Level 7, Inc. HL7 electronic health record: system functional model. Available at: www.hl7.org/EHR. Accessed March 19, 2007

8. Certification Commission for Healthcare Information Technology. Preparing for CCHIT certification. Available at: www.cchit.org/vendors/apply. Accessed February 20, 2007

9. Schillinger D, Piette J, Grumbach K, et al. Closing the loop: physician communication with diabetic patients who have low health literacy. *Arch Intern Med.* 2003;163:83–90

10. Chaudhry B, Wang J, Wu S, et al. Systematic review: impact of health information technology on quality, efficiency, and costs of medical care. *Ann Intern Med.* 2006;144:742–752

11. Dassenko D, Slowinski T. Using the CPR to benefit a business office. *Healthc Financ Manage.* 1995;49(7):68–70, 72–73

12. Embi PJ, Jain A, Clark J, Bizjack S, Hornung R, Harris CM. Effect of a clinical trial alert system on physician participation in trial recruitment. *Arch Intern Med.* 2005;165:2272–2277

13. Ford EW, Menachemi N, Phillips MT. Predicting the adoption of electronic health records by physicians: when will health care be paperless? *J Am Med Inform Assoc.* 2006;13:106–112

14. Kemper AR, Uren RL, Clark SJ. Adoption of electronic health records in primary care pediatric practices. *Pediatrics.* 2006;118(1). Available at: www.pediatrics.org/cgi/content/full/118/1/e20

15. Renner K, Renner K. Cost-justifying electronic medical records. *Healthc Financ Manage.* 1996;50(10):63–64

16. Ash JS, Berg M, Coiera E. Some unintended consequences of information technology in health care: the nature of patient care information system-related errors. *J Am Med Inform Assoc.* 2004;11:104–112

17. Schmitt KF, Wofford DA. Financial analysis projects clear returns from electronic medical records. *Healthc Financ Manage.* 2002;56(1):52–57

18. Adams WG, Mann AM, Bauchner H. Use of an electronic medical record improves the quality of urban pediatric primary care. *Pediatrics.* 2003;111:626–632

19. Spooner SA; American Academy of Pediatrics, Council on Clinical Information Technology. Special requirements of electronic health record systems in pediatrics. *Pediatrics.* 2007;119:631–637

20. Leavitt M, O'Kane ME. Joint statement from the National Commission for Quality Assurance and the Certification Commission for Health Care and Information Technology. Available at: www.ncqa.org/communications/Joint%20Statement%20on%20EHR%20Cert%20Rev%203%20_2_.pdf. Accessed July 16, 2003

21. New York City Department of Health and Mental Hygiene. Mayor Bloomberg proposes sweeping changes in health care financing through new use of information technology and new focus on prevention [press release]. Available at: www.nyc.gov/html/doh/html/pr2007/mr048-07.shtml. Accessed March 17, 2007

22. Eaton DK, Kann L, Kinchen S, et al. Youth risk behavior surveillance: United States, 2005. *MMWR Surveill Summ.* 2006;55(5):1–108

23. Klein JD, Wilson KM. Delivering quality care: adolescents' discussion of health risks with their providers. *J Adolesc Health.* 2002;30:190–195

24. Merenstein D, Green L, Fryer GE, Dovey S. Shortchanging adolescents: room for improvement in preventive care by physicians. *Fam Med.* 2001;33:120–123

25. Blum RW, Beuhring T, Wunderlich M, Resnick MD. Don't ask, they won't tell: the quality of adolescent health screening in five practice settings. *Am J Public Health.* 1996;86:1767–1772

26. Department of Adolescent Health. *Guidelines for Adolescent Preventive Services (GAPS) Recommendations Monograph.* Chicago, IL: American Medical Association; 1997

27. Society for Adolescent Medicine. Access to health care for adolescents and young adults. *J Adolesc Health.* 2004;35:342–344

Adolesc Med 18 (2007) 256–270

Office-Based Computerized Risk-Assessment and Health-Education Systems

David M. N. Paperny, MD, FAAP, FSAM*

Adolescent Clinic, Kaiser Permanente, and Department of Pediatrics, University of Hawaii School of Medicine, 1010 Pensacola Street, Honolulu, HI 96814-2120, USA

Risky adolescent health behaviors cause enormous personal suffering and are expensive for our health care system. Proven clinical interventions and effective preventive services improve adolescent health and reduce the personal and societal costs. Clinicians repeatedly interview patients and provide health advice, with variable efficacy and large investments in clinical time. Computer-assisted health evaluation of an adolescent's needs and problems can enhance the timeliness and reliability of health services. Patient-assessment software and health-education multimedia are readily available clinical tools.

Adolescent and young adult morbidity (and mortality) is mostly the consequence of preventable risk behaviors.[1] With the increasing importance of delivering preventive services and interventions to adolescents at risk, both parents and adolescents ask health care providers to address a broader range of services during clinical encounters.[2–5] Technology that allows health providers to easily have useful behavioral and medical information at their fingertips facilitates improved access, prevention, and health education. Such technology helps health providers make sounder medical decisions, facilitates personalized advice, and improves case management.

IMPROVED PREVENTION, PERSONALIZED INTERVENTIONS, AND POPULATION MANAGEMENT

Many approaches to identify high-risk adolescents, provide health education, prevent behaviors with poor outcomes, and promote professional intervention have had limited success.[6] A major obstacle to intervention in the medical setting is the personal sensitivity of these issues, which creates avoidance, discomfort,

---

*Corresponding author.
E-mail address: dpaperny@aol.com (D. M. N. Paperny).
Financial Disclosure: Dr Paperny is an officer and content creator for HealthMedia Corp, developer of the Youth Health Program.

and confidentiality concerns. The low rate of "sensitive" services provided to adolescents has also been attributed to clinicians' "forgetfulness."[7] Screening questionnaires, computerized health assessments, and computerized prompting systems have all helped to improve services for adolescents at risk.[8–10]

An early health-history–taking computer program was created on a mainframe computer at the University of California San Francisco Adolescent Clinic.[11] Comparing a mainframe computer terminal, a self-administered questionnaire, and a face-to-face interview, researchers in the early 1980s interviewed 108 adolescent girls about their sexual behavior. These young women preferred and were more comfortable with the computer interview method, finding it "fun," "private," "easy," and "interesting." This automated interview method was validated as an acceptable way to collect accurate sexual history information from adolescent girls, but the program gave no automated feedback. The University of Wisconsin's Barny program was designed with an interactive gaming format and was the first interactive computer-based health-education system for adolescents.[12]

Interactive health guidance with adolescents is always more effective than simply providing factual information, but it is more time consuming. Technology can aid health care providers to identify health-risk behaviors and help adolescents evaluate the consequences of their behavioral choices. Interactive multimedia allows confidentiality and provides developmentally appropriate, gender- and race-specific health education to teens. Computerized educational feedback can be generated from health-history questions, and associations between responses can be evaluated by an expert system. The resulting individualized simulations and personalized feedback can enhance higher-level interventions that would usually be too time consuming and even impractical in many clinical settings.

To deliver more cost-effective services to the adolescent population, creative use of automation can expand the capacity of the health care system.[13] Allied health professionals and paraprofessionals, along with use of educational technology, can expand our capacity to deliver a more full range of services to the many adolescents at risk.[14] Early detection and risk assessment with personalized interventions are essential for managing adolescent health issues. Routine anticipatory health guidance should be provided by a variety of methods and media (eg, health-education groups, audiovisual materials, referral to trusted Internet sites, and computer-based interactive multimedia).[7]

The paradigm shift in adolescent medicine from the traditional intervention/disease model to a health-promotion/prevention model has included an emphasis on targeted social/behavioral morbidities and a de-emphasis on biomedical problems alone. Technology helps providers to easily shift focus from prevention to intervention when the need arises and to prioritize interventions on the basis of problem severity and efficacy of the treatment approach. Many insurance payers and health plans either provide or require the use of certain computer software systems. These systems must include the functionality of automated screening and health-risk appraisal (HRA) systems, as well as education and training.[15]

HEALTH SCREENING AND ASSESSMENT

The personal health interview with counseling can be simulated by expert interactive multimedia software systems, which use complex rule-based algorithms for branching and decision-making.[16] The algorithms depend on the adolescent's responses, which control output and feedback. This automated process minimizes interpersonal barriers such as avoidance, discomfort, denial, and confidentiality concerns. An automated screening-interview assessment can be done by telephone automation (press a number or speak a response), by Internet, or at a personal computer or network terminal. The mechanism of information input is inconsequential to the information flow, validity of data collected, and appropriate educational feedback generated. An interactive screening of college students for hepatitis B used an automated telephone interview followed by selective referral to the college health service for those who were at risk and needed vaccination.[17]

Progress in the Computer-Assisted Self-Interview

Adolescents are drawn to new technology. An objective computer program designed to generate a health assessment that is accurate and personalized naturally attracts this population.[12,18] In previous studies, youth have indicated that, for sensitive topics, they prefer interactive computer interviews and training programs over direct human interventions. Of equal importance, it has been demonstrated that adolescents freely reveal sensitive information to computers.[11,19,20]

Early, comprehensive research on adolescents and computer-assisted self-interview (CASI) technology compared 3 matched groups: (1) 265 anonymous computer users; (2) a group of 294 computer users who were predirected to share a printout of their responses with a clinician; and (3) a group of 240 participants who completed written questionnaires and shared them.[9] The surveys included questions on sexual behavior, interest in contraceptive information, and adjustment/emotional issues. Both of the computer groups (anonymous versus shared) were comparable in sensitivity and better at detecting sensitive issues than the written questionnaire.

Additional assessments of teen opinion and self-report on the computer interview process included 4266 first-time users (3276 teens in medical clinic settings, 640 in public health fair settings, and 288 in detention, runaway shelters, or youth corrections facility, aged 13–19 years [mean: 15.5 years]; 54% female).[21] Because the evaluation was conducted before results were printed, responses were reflective only of the questioning, not the automated feedback. When the program asked, "How honest and accurate have you been with me on these questions?" teens responded 85% of the time that they were totally honest and accurate, 8% that they were not completely honest, 5% that they could not understand some of it, and 2% that they were pretty inaccurate. The computer was preferred by 89% of the respondents, whereas only 5% preferred a personal interview and 6% preferred a paper-based questionnaire interview. When asked, "How did you like talking to the computer?" 85% responded positively, 12% responded neutrally, and 3% responded negatively. On a 1-to-5 Likert scale (3, neutral; 5, high), the overall rating of the interview was 4.35.

In a subgroup of 200 teens, 97% responded that they gave their real and true information, 96% felt that the questions were appropriate, 95% reported that they read the printed feedback, and 97% felt that the results applied to them. When asked if they would like to use the computer again sometime, 87% responded affirmatively. Data from a separate group of 995 repeat users showed only 3% more respondents claiming dishonest answers and 4% fewer liking the computer.

CASI technology has also been tested on adolescents in acute crises and with specialty needs. In 2 particular instances, a CASI was used to evaluate sexual abuse history among adolescents in general and also in homeless youth.[22,23] The confidential computer interview detected sexual abuse, printed appropriate medical advice and resources, directed each abused teen to speak to the doctor or a parent about the abuse, and printed referrals to the local sexual abuse helpline. The most important conclusion these studies and experiences suggest is that divulging sensitive information to health personnel is not a problem; indeed, teens want to talk, but the "nonpersonal" method of obtaining the information protects them from embarrassment and perceived judgment.

CASI Functionality Enhanced With Multimedia

It is clear that automated health screening and assessment can use expert computer software to take general medical and behavioral histories, which can comfortably prime a face-to-face interview with health information. For patients, it can be fun, easy, and interesting and can enhance privacy and feedback reliability if it provides automated medical advice and referral. Clearly, adolescents are more comfortable and honest with the computer about sensitive behavioral health information.

Automated interview assessments accomplish a health evaluation by proceeding logically in the history-taking format of a trained clinician. They use complex relational algorithms and built-in clinical logic validations to assess health risks and behaviors; then, as a result of responses, they can administer educational multimedia. Such a rule-based, interactive branching program accomplishes a directed history on the basis of screening questions and previous answers; some adolescents are asked a minimum of screening questions, whereas others are asked more on the basis of individualized responses that require a more in-depth pathway of exploration. Internal cross-validation of responses for consistency and the opportunity to backtrack to clarify answers maximizes specificity of the interview.

Currently, only the Youth Health Program provides feedback including interactive, personalized multimedia presentations.[9,21,24] This feedback is followed by printed information with specific health advice as well as referrals to health resources. The system also conserves professional time when the clinician is given the printed problem list, which is based on the adolescent's interview responses.[14] It has been used in clinics, schools, community agencies, and other settings as part of a health evaluation visit with a clinician or counselor and as a stand-alone assessment and educational tool at kiosks, health fairs, and education centers (self-service mode, requiring no supervision). Although the software is self-service and anonymous, it invites (and repeatedly suggests that) the youth share results with the clinician or health educator. The program internally validates responses for consistency with previous screening responses and reconfirms crucial branch-point questions, which maximizes specificity. The interactive, multimedia presentations of the Youth Health Program are culturally diverse; each youth who uses the program, after answering questions about his or her gender and racial background, will have assessment questions and educational materials delivered by videos of culturally similar youths, which maximizes rapport and credibility.

Applications of CASI

Recommendations for content and delivery of preventive services for adolescents including *The Guidelines for Adolescent Preventive Services (GAPS)*[25] and *Bright Futures, Guidelines for Health Supervision of Infants, Children, and Adolescents*[26] emphasize behavioral and psychological components and de-emphasize screening for biomedical problems. Such screening and counseling for problem behaviors is time intensive. Although the outcome effectiveness of comprehensive adolescent preventive services is currently under study,[27] research to this point suggests that even limited behavioral change and risk reduction has profound long-term effects on the lives of adolescents.[28,29]

One application of CASI was with a low-cost team strategy to provide preventive health services to adolescents using computerized health assessments with individualized educational videos, trained health counselors, and nurses.[14] At sites including schools and shopping malls, adolescents completed confidential computerized health assessments, received individualized feedback, and viewed automated multimedia on a laptop computer. The computer also printed a prioritized problem list for a graduate-student–level health counselor to review with the adolescent. A registered nurse performed additional counseling when indicated.

On average, respondents spent 21 minutes completing the automated health assessment and viewing interactive multimedia and 15 minutes with the health counselor (range: 3–30 minutes). A vast majority (98%) had ≥1 risk behavior identified (see Table 1). One third required additional evaluation and counseling by the nurse (average 8 minutes). Educators reported that they felt only 3% of the youths were uncomfortable discussing sensitive issues, and only 5% of the youths asked about confidentiality. Discussions documented by educators were comparable in content to those reported by subjects on exit questionnaires. More than 90% of the patients were satisfied with the time spent.

Cost analysis revealed that a team of 2 computers, 2 counselors, and 1 nurse provided comprehensive screening and health counseling to 1 patient every 10 minutes at a salary cost of $7.46 per visit. The projected net cost (including training, administration, and turnover) was $15 per visit, approximately one fifth of the cost of a physical conducted by a physician. Comparative evaluation of the CASI-paraprofessional model to demographically matched preventive physical visits with 16 pediatricians and family practitioners found that significantly more health problems were identified, addressed, and documented by the team than by the physicians in traditional settings.

Because the use of computers and paraprofessional health counselors was a feasible, economical, and innovative alternative to the routine physical examination, this model was modified for use at a large health maintenance organization in Hawaii. Five years of data suggested increased access to needed preventive services by adolescents at a very modest cost.[30] This new approach provided effective screening for health-compromising behaviors, individualized health education, and necessary physical examinations. Detected risks were comparable

Table 1
Identified risk behaviors (N = 258)

Behavior	%
Stress	45
Helmet nonuse	43
Sexual activity without contraception	36
Family issues	29
Alcohol use	18
Violence exposure	17
DUI/passenger of someone else DUI	15
Poor communication skills	14
Seatbelt nonuse	14
Major affective issues	11
Significant suicide risk	3
Sexual abuse history	3
Physical abuse history	2

DUI indicates driving under the influence.

to those of previous studies. The adapted program identified several health risks including suicidal ideation and alcohol abuse. The respondents were split between liking the program (59%) and having no opinion (40%). A large majority (91%) felt that the program was just the right length.

Computer-assisted assessment of health needs and risks is thorough, accurate, painless, and easy and saves interviewer time. Automated screening and appraisal of health problems is interactive (expert interview via computer, telephone, or Internet) and can easily surface sensitive problems. It expedites accurate clinical assessments by reducing interview time and promotes quality care, because the clinician is preloaded with information from standardized interview questions. A CASI can alert those adolescents who may be unaware that they need health education or services. With associated multimedia, CASI facilitates acceptance and retention of health concepts, increases understanding of problem management and self-help, and may result in lower-risk health behaviors and improved compliance.

HRA Databases

When HRAs are downloaded as data from a computerized screening interview, a diagnostic problem list can be assembled. The database is primarily used to collect and organize the data on patients so that practitioners and educators can track those adolescents who need case management. Ticklers, provider alerts, and reminders can be automatically generated. Such a database often includes patients identified with affective issues, abuse, contraception and sexually transmitted disease issues, substance abuse, safety issues, and chronic medical conditions. At a clinic visit or by query, a summary report of an adolescent's current risks and clinical compliance can be made.

Research Applications

Because clinicians may deal with a wide range of issues during encounters, aggregate data can be made available for outcomes research.[7] Such a study that evaluated the effects of a preventive-services intervention on adolescent behavior showed that adolescents who received preventive services reported lower rates of risky behaviors compared with those in a baseline sample. These results suggest that screening and counseling for specific health-risk behaviors may favorably influence adolescent behavior.[27]

The screening-interview database enables comprehensive study of interrelationships between health and behavioral risks within and between adolescent populations. Using statistical programs, a provider or clinic can evaluate the practice and then provide more focused informational materials to specific patient groups (eg, early drug experimenters or adolescents who need contraception) for which early interventions are effective.

Patient Privacy and Confidentiality Issues

For a reliable computerized screening interview, it is necessary to provide complete privacy. There may be a perception by a few adolescents of lack of confidentiality in various settings, and some ask if their information is being electronically transmitted elsewhere. Certain branching-interview programs allow adolescents to control whether selected sensitive information is or is not disclosed to the clinician. Nevertheless, it will provide pertinent feedback and multimedia to the adolescent on those secure areas.

TECHNOLOGY-ASSISTED HEALTH EDUCATION

Every opportunity should be used to identify high-risk adolescents while administering and reinforcing health-promotion messages. Because clinical outcomes can be optimized, we can serve patients best by offering them health education using the media with which they are most familiar: television, video, and computers. We normally speak to adolescents to communicate medical advice, but understanding, acceptance, assimilation, and retention of verbal advice varies widely, as does patient compliance with health recommendations.[31] The usual written instructions and printed brochures are often provided and discarded, but we can now use technology that constitutes far more acceptable and effective patient education. Because cognitive services and health education are time intensive, health providers and clinics should consider information technology and use of specialized paraprofessional manpower for producing practical and cost-effective clinical outcomes. Appropriate combinations of allied health personnel, health educators, and peer counselors working with information technology discussed earlier in this chapter offer a potent intervention approach to adolescent health promotion in various settings.[14]

The Foundation of Multimedia: Video

Video is nearly ubiquitous for adolescents worldwide. In Spain, a survey of 884 teens revealed that 24% of families with teens had ≥4 television sets at home.[32] In youths' rooms, 53% had televisions, 58% had computers, and 52% had Internet access. Health professionals should take advantage of these technologies currently in the hands of adolescents to promote health education.

Clinicians and educators give guidance by repeating daily the same standardized health information to adolescents, and there is increasing demand to use video and multimedia as adjuncts to the spoken and printed word. Surveys suggest that patient-education videos are desired by both clinicians and patients in >80% of office visits.[33] However, according to some American Academy of Pediatrics surveys, <20% of pediatricians use patient-education videos during office visits. Feedback in clinical studies of patient-education videos suggests that patients are receptive and find succinct presentations to be quite helpful.[33]

Routine video use in clinical settings is usually limited by a number of obstacles: the nonstandard paradigm, patient flow and space limitations, and limited materials; most existing videos are long and inefficient, have not been tested by the target population for effect, lack simple layman's language to ensure comprehension, and do not use "television-quality" production to hold viewer attention. For practical office use, a video topic must be short and powerfully presented.

Perhaps the most important use of health-education video is to teach basic concepts and allow professionals to more efficiently focus their time on evaluating patient understanding and obstacles to behavior change. In addition, the video scripts can be uniquely precise medical record documentation.

Direct video reinforcement of a clinician's advice is another useful adjunct to enhance retention and improve compliance. Studies have shown that youth retain greater amounts of knowledge when watching a screen than listening to a person and that compliance with medical directives can increase by as much as 50%.[34,35] Video can enable clinicians to more thoroughly demonstrate health behaviors and home management techniques, visually show the danger signs that patients should watch for when sick, and validate medical advice for skeptical adolescents.[36]

When videos are to be obtained and used for health education, the health provider or educator must be aware of criteria for evaluation of patient-education video productions when incorporating and using them in the clinical setting. The characteristics of quality video are:

- concise 1- to 3-minute video format that holds adolescents' attention and will not obstruct examination rooms or patient flow;
- succinct, understandable programs that emphasize main points and give the priority advice;
- meticulous script wording designed to be understandable, nontechnical, timeless, and universal while avoiding conjecture, controversy, and bias;
- captivating and timeless images that reinforce the main points of a voice-over spoken message;
- warm close-ups with good lighting and frequent scene changes (approximately every 3–4 seconds);
- appropriate computer-generated diagrams or lettering;
- camera angles that avoid a recognizable clinician, providing a custom-produced look; and
- no extended talking heads or lectures.

Administration of Video in Medical Settings

In the busy medical setting, it is not practical to use cumbersome videotapes, which require rewinding to search for topics and eventually wear out. Current digital compact videodisks eliminate these problems. The format called video-CD (VCD) is simpler than DVD, and the VCD video files can be shown on any examination room computer terminal used for HRA or even an electronic medical record.

Simple innovative applications of now-common technology can overcome many of the current obstacles to clinical communication with adolescents. Enhanced outcomes can result from routinely educating at-risk youths using the media with which they are most familiar. As more adolescent-directed content and products become available, and more clinicians and educators produce well-developed and tested video vignettes, video-enhanced health promotion should become a routine adjunct in the clinical setting. The technical advantages and disadvantages of using VCDs and DVDs in adolescent health education are listed in Table 2.

Progress in the Use of Video Media and DVD in Health Education

Numerous applications of video used in training and health education have been successful, but until now, it has been impractical for busy emergency departments caring for adolescents to routinely use educational video because of high patient flow.[37,38] An emergency department demonstration project[39] used immediate asthma training with an interactive, branching DVD[40] to teach asthma care skills, often while adolescents received a nebulizer treatment. Sound provided via headphones for the patient and parent and succinct presentations were designed to allow for continued patient flow. Most new patients had a standard 15-minute vignette with a pretest and posttest. Topics were age specific for children, adolescents, or adults. For return patients, the clinician wrote prescriptions to

Table 2
Pros and cons of video education

VCD in Adolescent Health Education	DVD in Adolescent Health Education
Advantages	Advantages
Up to 99 video segments	Unlimited video segments
Lowest production, duplication, and revision costs	MEPG-2 (and above) is a higher-quality video format and very clear
MPEG-1–level video format can be stored/shown as computer files	Authoring allows branching and interactive programming
Disadvantages	Disadvantages
Format may not play on all DVD players	Must be shown from a DVD disk, not a computer file
Limited level of interactivity; no branching	Higher duplication and revision costs
MPEG-1 lower-level format is VHS-quality video	Total production and authoring is more complex and costly
Video clips must meet the same quality editing standards as DVD	

show a shorter course with selected additional subjects by using preprinted "asthma video Rx" forms. Physicians could prescribe additional relevant DVD video selections to any patient when clinically indicated. The asthma care DVD branched through 19 age-specific topics for infants (0–5 years), children/youths (5–14 years), and young adults (>15 years). Testing and follow-up showed that patient compliance and asthma care skills were enhanced by supplementing emergency department treatments with video health education.

Similar positive results of multimedia-enhanced patient-education projects were found for smoking cessation via the Internet,[41] breast self-examination for high school girls,[42] and parental awareness of fever in children and adolescents.[43]

As programs have expanded, concerns about cost have as well. The common DVD offers a uniquely flexible, low-cost option with a wide range of training possibilities. Conservative projections of medical cost and resource savings suggest that health promotion resulting in even small percentages of behavior change and morbidity reduction can have profound and significant long-term effects on entire populations of adolescents. To be cost-effective, preventive educational services may only need to eliminate 5% to 15% of morbidities.[28]

Computer-Assisted Instruction: The Precursor to Interactive Multimedia

Experiential computer programs can act as mediators to facilitate mature, informed decision-making by adolescents who need not suffer the embarrassment or actual consequences of poor health choices. Risk-taking and reality-testing by adolescents may be modified by automated choice assessment in combination with directed educational feedback, giving them better decision-making information. Adolescents enjoy animated-action, color computer games and training software that capture and hold their attention by using problem-solving situations, simulations, and scenarios. Game-format computer-assisted instruction algorithms can be powerful health-education tools that use an interactive/responsive format, provide information, and simulate outcomes, creating the impact of reality. Adolescents actively explore health alternatives, outcomes, and their consequences in games. Interactive educational activities can modify adolescent health behaviors by sharing knowledge, correcting misconceptions, and allowing adolescents to practice desired behaviors and appropriate decision-making skills. These media have also been shown to reduce counseling time and facilitate acceptance and retention of critical health concepts.[44]

Interactive Patient Health-Education Multimedia

There are a number of different kinds of interactive multimedia, including Laserdisc level 3 (now obsolete), interactive digital video (minimally, VCD; maximally, DVD), the computer CD-ROM, media retrieval (some on Internet), and distance learning (some also on the Internet). Interactive multimedia technology that provides automated health education and age-specific anticipatory guidance can be very credible, give prioritized and confidential information, and save clinician time.

Determining Quality and Usability of Multimedia for Clinical Application

Significant amounts of time and funding are often spent on technology with suboptimal results because of poor program evaluation, inadequate administrative preplanning, and incorrect needs assessment. The presentation criteria for multimedia are:

- clarity and ease of use;
- appeal of presentation;
- color and graphics quality and usefulness;
- audio effects and enhancement; and
- language style and timing.

Operational considerations for determining the usefulness of multimedia are:
- branching ability of program choices and interview techniques;
- instructional value;
- accuracy of information and content;
- personalized feedback provided on the basis of input;
- instructional formats used;
- time required to finish (average: 25 minutes); and
- documentation and support for the larger program.

The adolescent health provider should assess potential health-education and assessment programs before incorporating and using one. Additional information on what to look for and how to assess the material has been outlined elsewhere.[45]

STATE-OF-THE-ART CLINICAL ENCOUNTER

In this scenario, an adolescent presents at a medical office and then sits at a terminal located in the waiting room, where he or she completes his or her screening interview on a touchpad. This expert system uses complicated branching logic to elicit medical, health, and behavioral history relevant to the visit. The adolescent chooses whether he or she is seeing the clinician for a sick visit or a health appraisal and covers updates of specific problem areas previously known about him or her from the office HRA database. Using earphones, the adolescent may watch a clinic information video (personalized by the clinician) or health-information vignettes regarding the assessed chief complaint (eg, acne management). He or she is brought into an examination room to finish the expert screening interview or health-education videos on the examination room monitors.

This youth is now on the patient record screen of the clinician's office-pad portable workstation, which shows the download of his or her screening interview. The clinician reviews the prioritized concerns and automated assessment obtained from the patient. After examination, in response to the patient's questions, the doctor selects on his or her portable workstation's screen a number of patient-education materials (including specific diagnosis-related videos) and patient-personalized handouts to be printed. He or she receives interactive multimedia training ordered on other adolescent topics. The office health-education system has digital video/DVD servers with office-wide closed-circuit distribution nodes. The office visit is completely video-recorded (physician in the examination room with the adolescent and all the explanations given, as well as every health-education video prescribed) both for patient review and relevant family if not there, as well as for medicolegal documentation. This is recorded onto DVD to take home. At patient sign-out, the office system prints future appointments, handouts, and patient instructions.

EMERGING TECHNOLOGIES

Integration of health screening and education materials with larger information systems and electronic medical records is usually via a "server network," where information is available for many functional areas. Total integration of the separate electronic systems will provide timely access to information.[46] As improved integration of information systems occurs, an amazing array of medical and health-information technology will potentially interact seamlessly to create an efficient, convenient, and efficacious health screening and education system previously unheard of in health care.[45]

How far can the future of health screening and education take us? There is now a plethora of modes of sharing information in many formats, and most adolescents are well wired. Many teens are now using cell-phone units that have photograph and text messaging, MP3 (music and sound), videos, still and video cameras, calendar reminders, alarms, and Internet service. Podcasts are a new form of sharing video and high-bandwidth information.

Advertisers pay huge sums to get the "attention" of adolescents and young adults. We need to seriously consider incentives to health education and promote positive health messages for adolescents and young adults via these new media. Repetitive violent and negative messages, such as certain television, music, and computer games, must be replaced by positive content. When technology is used to promote healthy choices and attitudes (with safeguards to eliminate concerns about privacy), we allow all of our technologically advanced youth to engage in their own health on many levels.

REFERENCES

1. Haggerty RJ. The new morbidity. In: Haggerty RJ, Roghmann KJ, Pless IB, eds. *Child Health and Community*. New York, NY: Wiley; 1975:1–12

2. Fisher M. Parents' views of adolescent health issues. *Pediatrics*. 1992;90:335–341
3. Joffe A, Radius S, Gall M. Health counseling for adolescents: what they want, what they get, and who gives it. *Pediatrics*. 1988;82:481–485
4. Millstein SG. A view of health from the adolescent's perspective. In: Millstein SG, Petersen AC, Nightingale EO, eds. *Promoting the Health of Adolescents: New Directions for the Twenty-first Century*. New York, NY: Oxford University Press; 1993:97–118
5. Sobal J, Klein H, Graham D, Black J. Health concerns of high school students and teachers' beliefs about student health concerns. *Pediatrics*. 1988;81:218–223
6. McAnarney ER. Discontinuity: a dilemma for adolescents. *Pediatrics*. 1987;80:954–956
7. Rosen D, Elster A, Hedberg V, Paperny D. Clinical preventive services for adolescents: position paper of the Society for Adolescent Medicine. *J Adolesc Health*. 1997;21:203–214
8. Schubiner H, Tzelepis A, Wright K, Podany E. The clinical utility of the Safe Times Questionnaire. *J Adolesc Health*. 1994;15:374–382
9. Paperny DM, Aono JY, Lehman RM, Hammar SL, Risser J. Computer-assisted detection and intervention in adolescent high-risk health behaviors. *J Pediatr*. 1990;116:456–462
10. Litzelman DK, Dittus RS, Miller ME, Tierney WM. Requiring physicians to respond to computerized reminders improves their compliance with preventive care protocols. *J Gen Intern Med*. 1993;8:311–317
11. Millstein S, Irwin C. Acceptability of computer-acquired sexual histories in adolescent girls. *J Pediatr*. 1983;103:815–819
12. Bosworth K, Gustafson DH, Hawkins RP, Chewning B, Day T. Adolescents, health education, and computers: the Body Awareness Resource Network (BARN). *Health Educ*. 1983;14:58–60
13. Elster AB. Confronting the crisis in adolescent health: visions for change. *J Adolesc Health*. 1993;14:505–508
14. Paperny DM, Hedberg V. Computer-assisted health counselor visits: a low-cost model for comprehensive adolescent preventive services. *Arch Pediatr Adolesc Med*. 1999;153:63–67
15. Paperny DM, Zurhellen W, Lighter D, et al. W312: the pediatric office: 2000 and beyond [workshop]. Presented at: the American Academy of Pediatrics annual meeting; October 11, 1999; Washington, DC
16. Rathbun J. Development of a computerized alcohol screening instrument for the university community. *J Am Coll Health*. 1993;42:33–36
17. Havel RD, Wright MP. Automated interviewing for hepatitis B risk assessment and vaccination referral. *Am J Prev Med*. 1997;13:392–395
18. Chen M. How effective are microcomputer-based programs for health education: a prospective view. *Health Educ*. 1983;14:88–89
19. Slack WV. Computer-based interviewing system dealing with nonverbal behavior as well as keyboard responses. *Science*. 1971;171:84–87
20. Fisher LA, Johnson TS, Porter D, Bleich HL, Slack WV. Collection of a clean voided urine specimen: a comparison among spoken, written, and computer-based instructions. *Am J Public Health*. 1977;67:640–644
21. Paperny DM. Computerized health assessment and education for adolescent HIV and STD prevention in healthcare settings and schools. *Health Educ Behav*. 1997;24:54–70
22. Paperny DM, Aono JY, Lehman RM, Hammar SL. Computer-assisted detection, evaluation, and referral of sexually abused adolescents. *J Adolesc Health*. 1988;9:260
23. Johnson RJ, Rew L, Sternglanz RW. The relationship between childhood sexual abuse and sexual health practices of homeless adolescents. *Adolescence*. 2006;41:221–234
24. HealthMedia Corporation. Youth health program. Available at: http://healthmediacorp.com/_wsn/page2.html. Accessed February 1, 2007
25. Elster AB, Kuznets NJ. *AMA Guidelines for Adolescent Preventive Services (GAPS): Recommendations and Rationale*. Baltimore, MD: Williams and Wilkins; 1994
26. Green ME. *Bright Futures: Guidelines for Health Supervision of Infants, Children, and Adolescents*. Arlington, VA: National Center for Education in Maternal and Child Health; 1994
27. Ozer E, Adams S, Lustig J, et al. Clinical preventive services make a difference in adolescent behavior. *J Adolesc Health*. 2004;32:132

28. Gans JE, Alexander B, Chu RC, Elster AB. The cost of comprehensive preventive medical services for adolescents. *Arch Pediatr Adolesc Med.* 1995;149:1226–1234

29. Downs SM, Klein JD. Clinical preventive services efficacy and adolescents' risky behaviors. *Arch Pediatr Adolesc Med.* 1995;149:374–379

30. Adolescent Services Program. *5-Year Report 1998–2003: Youth Health Appraisal/Teen and Young Adult Checkup.* Honolulu, HI: Kaiser Permanente Hawaii Region; 2003

31. Bartlett EE. Effective approaches to patient education for the busy pediatrician. *Pediatrics.* 1984;74(5 pt 2):920–923

32. Bercedo Sanz A, Redondo Figuero C, Pelayo Alonso R, Gomez Del Rio Z, Hernandez Herrero M, Cadenas Gonzalez N. Mass media consumption in adolescence [in Spanish]. *An Pediatr (Barc).* 2005;63:516–525

33. Paperny DM. Pediatric medical advice enhanced with use of video. *Am J Dis Child.* 1992;146: 785–786

34. Paperny DM. Automated adolescent preventative services using computer-assisted video multimedia [abstract]. *J Adolesc Health.* 1994;15:66

35. Paperny DM. HMO innovations: video-enhanced medical advice. *HMO Pract.* 1991;5:212–213

36. Gagliano M. A literature review on the efficacy of video in patient education. *J Med Educ.* 1988;63:785–792

37. Marco CA, Larkin GL. Public education regarding resuscitation: effects of a multimedia intervention. *Ann Emerg Med.* 2003;42:256–260

38. Bynum AB, Cranford CO, Irwin CA, Denny GS. Participant satisfaction in an adult telehealth education program using interactive compressed video delivery methods in rural Arkansas. *J Rural Health.* 2003;19:218–222

39. Boychuk R, DeMesa C, Kiyabu K, et al. Change in approach and delivery of medical care in children with asthma: results from a multicenter emergency department educational asthma management program. *Pediatrics.* 2006;117(4 pt 2):S145–S151

40. HealthMedia Corp. The asthma care DVD: an interactive DVD to teach asthma care skills. Available at: http://healthmediacorp.com/_wsn/page2.html. Accessed February 1, 2007

41. Swartz LH, Noell JW, Schroeder SW, Ary DV. A randomised control study of a fully automated internet based smoking cessation programme. *Tob Control.* 2006;15:7–12

42. Ogletree RJ, Hammig B, Drolet JC, Birch DA. Knowledge and intentions of ninth-grade girls after a breast self-examination program. *J Sch Health.* 2004;74:365–369

43. Robinson JS, Schwartz ML, Magwene KS, Krengel SA, Tamburello D. The impact of fever health education on clinic utilization. *Am J Dis Child.* 1989;143:698–704

44. Krishna S, Balas EA, Spencer DC, Griffin JZ, Boren SA. Clinical trials of interactive computerized patient education: implications for family practice. *J Fam Pract.* 1997;45:25–33

45. Paperny DM, Zurhellen W, Spooner SA, et al. W415: advanced clinical computing strategies [workshop]. Presented at: the American Academy of Pediatrics annual meeting; October 12, 1999; Washington, DC

46. Zurhellen WM. The computerization of ambulatory pediatric practice. *Pediatrics.* 1995;96(4 pt 2):835–842; discussion 842–844

Adolesc Med 18 (2007) 271–292

Secure E-mail Applications: Strengthening Connections Between Adolescents, Parents, and Health Providers

Alwyn Cohall, MD*, Carly Hutchinson, MA, Andrea Nye, MPH

Harlem Health Promotion Center, Mailman School of Public Health, Columbia University, 215 West 125th Street, Ground Floor, New York, NY 10027, USA

Review of the literature suggests that electronic communication using e-mail can play an important role in improving the ability of adult consumers to connect with their health providers.[1,2] Similar potential may exist for this medium to strengthen connections between adolescents, their parents, and their health providers.[3] Here we summarize the advantages and limitations of electronic communication, review new developments in the field, and address specific issues germane to youth and their caregivers.

The average doctor's office or health clinic that serves adolescents and young adults is bombarded daily by youth or parents requesting appointments, prescription refills, and referrals to specialists, as well as information or advice on management of acute and chronic health concerns. Busy providers are constantly looking for strategies to make their practices more efficient and allow for more effective communication with patients and families. Similarly, young people and their parents are often searching for better ways to get their clinical and administrative needs met by health providers and their staff. Advances in technology may provide valuable assistance in facilitating these communication linkages between providers and their clientele.

Healthy People 2010 has acknowledged that:

> many health care organizations and public service agencies already use the Internet as one of their main channels for information dissemination. Access to the Internet and subsequent technologies is likely to become essential to gain access to health information, contact health organizations and health professionals, receive services at a distance, and participate in efforts to improve local and national health.[4]

---

*Corresponding author.
E-mail address*: atc1@columbia.edu (A. Cohall).

Increasingly, Americans are becoming connected to the Internet and logging on for a variety of purposes, including entertainment, education, networking, and communication.[5]

Adolescents are leading the way. Eighty-seven percent of all teenagers between the ages of 12 and 17 use the Internet, as compared with 66% of adults. Fifty-one percent say they go online at least once daily, and 21% report going online 3 to 5 times each week. Of adolescent Internet users, 89% use the Internet to send or read e-mail, 31% search for general health information, and 22% specifically find the Internet helpful in getting information on sensitive health topics such as drug use, sexual health, or depression.[6] The act of searching for health information reflects a natural curiosity on the part of young people who are trying to make sense of their changing bodies, feelings, and social contexts. It may also reflect the fact that many adolescents have limited contact with health providers[7] and, therefore, may need to seek additional sources of information to address their concerns. Furthermore, even when adolescents do present for a medical evaluation, opportunities are often missed for provision of information, advice, and counseling because of time constraints, parental presence, and provider discomfort.[8]

Similarly, studies suggest that parents, in general, desire more information and guidance on child rearing.[9] However, the average well-child encounter is only ~15 minutes,[10] and only 15% to 20% of parents recall their child's provider discussing psychosocial issues with them.[9] Parents of adolescents may be at an even greater disadvantage, given that adolescents make fewer visits to health providers than infants or children.[7] Likewise, parents may not accompany an adolescent to a visit because of work or other family obligations. Arguably, given the risk-taking potential for many adolescents, it seems that at a time when parents may need more advice and support from health providers, less is available. Technology has the potential to significantly enhance communication between providers and their clientele, thus helping to meet the needs of both doctors and their patients.

POTENTIAL ADVANTAGES OF E-MAIL COMMUNICATIONS

From the point of view of the consumer, encounters with any aspect of the health care system, whether private or public, can be potentially exasperating. Most primary care clinical settings operate during "normal" business hours when adolescents are in school or parents are at work or handling other childcare responsibilities. Scheduling an appointment, obtaining a referral, requesting a prescription renewal, getting results of laboratory or radiograph studies, clarifying instructions, or getting an answer to a simple health question may entail making several telephone calls and leaving multiple messages before satisfactory resolution is achieved. Although this may tax the patience of any adult consumer, it may be particularly problematic for adolescents with limited frustration tolerance and multiple time demands. Busy providers and their staff express similar frustrations as they frantically attempt to keep pace with ringing telephones, beeping fax machines, and vibrating pagers.

E-mail offers many valuable options. In contrast to the telephone, which is a "synchronous" medium, meaning that both sender and receiver must be connected at the same time for communication to ensue, e-mail is an "asynchronous" medium that allows for a built-in lag time between the time a message is sent, received, and answered.[11] This allows users to access and respond to messages at their convenience, which has significant implications for nonurgent communications between consumers and providers in clinical practice. From the consumer perspective, routine requests for appointments, prescriptions, or referrals can be initiated at any location where the Internet can be accessed, at any time, without having to wait on the telephone for a person to pick up the call. The provider's office can collect requests during the course of the day and designate a time period to review and respond that is consistent with the ebb and flow of their typical office pattern. Triage systems can also be set up so that messages can be routed to the most appropriate member of the office, be it receptionist, office manager, nurse, or medical provider.

E-mail requests and responses are also self-documenting, which makes it easy to create a paper trail of communication between patients, the provider's office, and other entities such as pharmacies or referral sources. Hard copies of e-mails can be printed and placed in the appropriate section of the medical chart, thus lessening the likelihood of messages "falling through the cracks" in busy office settings. In addition, the quality of information recorded can be detailed and cumulative, thus reflecting an entire exchange about a given subject.[12] For example, an adolescent with recurrent abdominal pain or headaches can fill out a detailed symptom diary and e-mail it to the provider for review before the next scheduled visit. This record may help detect contributing factors and suggest possible interventions. It also can be printed and maintained in the patient's medical record for precise documentation of the exchange.

Consumers seem supportive of e-mail as a communication tool. A Harris Interactive survey reported in 2002 that 90% of US adults who used the Internet wanted to communicate with their physician online.[13] A more recent Harris survey found that 77% of adults would like reminders via e-mail from their doctors regarding medical visits or other types of regular care. Seventy-five percent of those surveyed would appreciate the chance to schedule a doctor's visit via the Internet.[14]

Electronic Communication and Parents

Although consumers, in general, express interest in using e-mail as a way to communicate with their providers, parents seem particularly invested in this modality. Surveys have indicated clearly that parents are connected to the Internet, view health-information seeking as an important activity, and desire better linkages to their child's health providers. Seventy percent of parents in the United States with children at home under the age of 18 use the Internet, compared with 53% of nonparents (adults who do not have minor children in the household).[15] Ninety-two percent of the parents cited sending or receiving e-mail as a frequent online activity, and 67% use the Internet to search for health or medical information, most often on behalf of their child.[15] In addition, compared with nonparents, online parents were more likely to discuss information they found on the Internet with their health providers.[15] Furthermore, in a recent study of parents in an integrated pediatric health care delivery system providing primary and subspecialty care, 74% of parents expressed interest in using e-mail to contact their child's provider's office for reasons similar to those outlined above, including obtaining information and test results, scheduling appointments, and discussing their child's symptoms. Overall, 80% of the parents felt that all pediatricians should use e-mail to communicate with parents, and 65% stated that they would be more likely to choose a pediatrician on the basis of access by e-mail.[16]

In another study, although only 15% of the parents reported previously communicating with their child's health provider by e-mail, close to 50% stated that they would like to have this option, and 75% would be interested in extending e-mail communications to include receiving periodic e-mail newsletters from the office on well-child care and general health care.[17] Finally, to improve coordination of care, parents accessing emergency department services value the potential for e-mail to give their primary care providers information about their child's visit.[18]

Clearly, parents of infants and children seem to support electronic communication. However, little is known about how parents of adolescents feel about using e-mail to communicate with their teen's providers or what concerns they might have about their teens using this modality in a confidential fashion. Available research has suggested that parents value providers as a source of information and support for themselves and their teens[19] and generally support provision of confidential communication.[20] By inference, we could assume that the many parents of adolescents would welcome e-mail communications, although additional research is necessary. Anecdotally, in our private practice with adolescents, parents readily embrace this tool and have not expressed concern about extending this privilege to their adolescents.

Electronic Communication and Adolescents

As noted earlier, adolescents readily embrace technology, and although many prefer text messaging and instant messaging in communication with peers, focus groups involving youth find that they prefer e-mail as a mechanism for talking to "old people" or institutions.[6] To our knowledge, there have been no formal studies evaluating the extent to which adolescents desire or make attempts to communicate with their health providers. However, we do know that adolescents want and need advice about their health and view health providers as trusted resources.[21]

Many young people are uncomfortable discussing sensitive subjects face-to-face with their physician, especially if a parent is present. In a study conducted by Valaitis and Ruta[22] that focused on school-based development in inner-city Ontario, Canada, youth reported feeling substantially decreased anxiety by communicating with adults via online messages rather than face-to-face or on the telephone. This anxiety in communicating with adults stemmed from concerns about being able to "measure up," to speak correctly, and convey information adequately. "Usually people get choked up over the [telephone] line. If you write it, it is easier to say things." Overall, youth felt an increased sense of capability when they communicated with adults over the Internet, as opposed to other traditional forms. Thus, it would seem that e-mail should be avidly embraced by both consumers (of all ages) and providers. Review of the literature, however, suggests that its potential has only been partially realized.

PROVIDER RELUCTANCE TO EMBRACE ONLINE COMMUNICATIONS AND BARRIERS TO USE

Despite consumer interest and expert support,[11,23] evidence suggests that the majority of physicians have been relatively slow to embrace e-mail as a means of communicating with their patients. A gap seems to exist between consumers' desire and what they actually receive. Kassirer described the current situation: "Many patients are beginning to use online communication and are dragging their doctors along."[24] Currently, 75% of physicians do not use e-mail or other forms of electronic messaging with their patients.[25] Only ~5% report doing so regularly. Specifically, with regard to pediatricians, 1 study indicated that 79% of pediatricians had no desire to communicate with their patients via e-mail.[26] A study of the American Academy of Pediatrics membership in 2002 revealed that only 14% were using e-mail to communicate with their patients. Barriers to use of e-mail included the belief that there are too few patients with e-mail access (34%), lack of provider interest in communicating via e-mail (38%), lack of office staff time (42%), concerns about privacy or confidentiality (45%), and lack of physician time (52%).[27] In addition to the items mentioned above, other provider surveys have revealed concerns about lack of reimbursement as an implementation barrier.[28] Although all of these issues are legitimate, we believe that the advantages of e-mail outweigh its limitations,[1,29,30] that proper use of protocols will increase efficiency,[11,24] and that recent advances in technology will allow providers to feel more comfortable in using this promising medium.[29]

STRATEGIES FOR ADDRESSING PROVIDER CONCERNS

Limited E-mail Access by Patients

Providers may underestimate the extent to which their patients have access to the Internet and desire to communicate via e-mail. As previously noted, the majority of American consumers have access to and use the Internet and e-mail and want to communicate with their health providers. Although a "digital divide" continues to exist, wherein more affluent families have better access to technology, available data suggest that the gap is rapidly closing because of the lower costs of computers and their perceived utility for educational purposes among low-income families.[15] Specifically, with respect to adolescents and their families, although 90% of teens from families who earn more than $30 000/year have access to the Internet at home, 73% of teens who reside in households in which the income level is under $30 000/year also have such access.[6] Providers should also keep in mind that many low-income youth and their families may have access to the Internet through work, school, libraries, and community centers.[21] In addition, interest among low-income consumers regarding use of the Internet for information about health issues and communication with health providers is high.[31] Therefore, it would seem prudent for providers to adjust their thinking accordingly.

Time

Time is a precious commodity that is often in short supply in most clinical settings. Providers are understandably reluctant to embrace any change that may increase workloads. Many of them harbor the perception that they will be deluged by e-mail queries, often inappropriate, to which they will have to spend countless hours sorting, sifting, and responding. In reality, studies suggest that these concerns are generally unfounded. For example, 1 study collected a total of 3007 patient-physician e-mail messages over 11 months as part of a randomized, controlled trial of a triage-based e-mail system in 2 primary care centers; 10% of the messages were randomly selected for review. A majority (82.8%) of the messages addressed a single issue. The most common message types included information updates to the physicians (41.4%), prescription-renewal requests (24.2%), health questions (13.2%), questions about test results (10.9%), referrals (8.8%), "other" (including thank you's and apologies) (8.8%), appointment requests (5.4%), requests for non–health-related information (4.8%), and billing questions (0.3%). Overall, messages were concise, formal, and medically relevant. Very few (5.1%) included sensitive content, and none included urgent messages. Less than half (43.2%) required a direct physician response and, instead, were handled by other staff members.[29]

Compensation

Two thirds of doctors say they would use e-mail, but only if they were paid for the time involved.[25] Potentially, if providers could receive compensation by consumers and/or insurance companies for time spent addressing issues via e-mail, then motivation to use this modality might increase. In a study of adult patients, 40% stated that they would be willing to pay for the service,[2] a sentiment echoed by parents, as well.[16] In its report *Crossing the Quality Chasm*, the Institute of Medicine suggested that "access to care should be provided over the Internet, by phone. . .in addition to face-to-face visits" and that "a 2 minute E-mail communication could meet many patient's needs more responsively and at a lower cost."[32] In response, there is interest in the potential of e-mail to improve communication, deliver preventive-care messages, and even address minor complaints. A *Current Procedural Terminology* code has been developed for online consultations, and selected insurance companies seem to be willing to provide reimbursement for patients using this service.

Legal Implications of E-mail Communication

Perhaps the thorniest area to address with respect to electronic communication is the range of legal issues that concern providers. To begin, it is critical for physicians to realize that e-mail is a tool to enhance communication with patients with whom the provider has an established relationship.[33] In the event of receipt of unsolicited e-mails from patients who are unknown to the practice, the provider has no obligation to provide recommendations or advice.[34] For established patients, confidentiality is an important consideration, because doctors have both ethical and legal responsibilities to maintain the privacy and confidentiality of their communications about health information with and about their patients. General security regulations for e-mail communications that contain a patient's protected health information (PHI) are laid out in the Health Insurance Portability and Accountability Act (HIPAA), which was passed in 1996 to protect the privacy and security of health care information and to promote more standardization and efficiency in health care. Its provisions require health care providers, plans, and programs to handle all medical record transactions carefully and ensure specifically delineated privacy and security requirements. With respect to e-mail:

> The HIPAA Security Rule does not expressly prohibit the use of e-mail for sending electronic protected health information (PHI). However, the standards for access control (45 CFR §164.312(a)), integrity (45 CFR §164.312(c)(1)), and transmission security (45 CFR §164.312(e)(1)) require covered entities to implement policies and procedures to restrict access to, protect the integrity of, and guard against the unauthorized access to electronic PHI. The standard for transmission security (§164.312(e)) also includes addressable specifications for integrity controls and encryption. This means that the covered entity must assess its use of open networks, identify the available and appropriate means to protect electronic PHI as it is transmitted, select a solution, and document the decision. The Security Rule allows for electronic PHI to be sent over an electronic open network as long as it is adequately protected.[35]

Guidelines set forth by the American Medical Association (AMA)[36] and the American Medical Informatics Association (AMIA)[11] have also provided important parameters for physicians and their staffs when developing e-mail communication protocols with patients (see Table 1). Although these guidelines provide important direction, the extent to which they are used seems to be erratic. In 1 study, among those providers using e-mail to communicate with their patients, <7% complied with at least 7 of the 13 guidelines for e-mail communication.[33] Difficulties in complying with these guidelines may lay partially in the logistic problems inherent in the interface between office practice flow and standard e-mail systems.

Although there are many advantages to using e-mail, conventional systems are "unstructured and poorly designed for using forms for referrals and prescription renewals or for routing messages automatically. Lacking encryption, messages can be intercepted and read by prying eyes. And transferring messages into the patient's medical record can be awkward and time-consuming."[37]

In addition to the technical clumsiness of routing and responding appropriately and quickly to free-text messages generated by consumers, the security aspects of conventional e-mail lack the rigor required under HIPAA. The effectiveness of patient-provider electronic communications can be affected by both system- and individual-level failures. On the part of the system, for example, traditional servers offer limited protection against the alteration of e-mail messages, and although the sheer volume of transmission makes the probability low, it is still possible nonetheless. Encryption, the process of enhancing the fidelity of transmitting and receiving e-mail communications, provides a significant measure of security for both the sender and receiver of e-mail messages. However, until the advent of secure e-mail applications, the use of encryption software was expensive and cumbersome, thus potentially limiting the widespread use of e-mail in patient-provider communications.

On an individual level, if errors are made in the spelling of a user's e-mail account by the provider, the intended party may not receive an expected response, and the potential exists for complete strangers to receive confidential health information. E-mails sent to a home in which multiple individuals share a computer (and potentially passwords) may lead to inadvertent sharing of information. In addition, if a consumer fails to log off or leaves the computer screen unattended, information could be viewed by a third party.[30] This is of particular concern for adolescents, because 73% of teen users go online from a computer located in an open family space.[6] In addition, consumers may not realize that if they access the Internet at school or work, content of their e-mail messages may be subject to review by administrative officials. Thus, a number of logistic and security hurdles need to be overcome before the promise of electronic messaging becomes a viable adjunct to traditional forms of communication.

Table 1
Summary of AMA and AMIA guidelines for physician-patient electronic communications

Communications Guidelines	Medicolegal and Administrative Guidelines	Ethics Policy
General policies		
Inform patients about privacy issues such as who on the provider staff may be processing messages; procedure for addressing messages during vacations; and that messages will become part of their medical record	Develop patient-clinician agreement for informed consent for the use of e-mail	E-mail should not be used to establish a patient-physician relationship; rather, it should supplement more personal encounters; medical advice or information specific to the patient's condition should not be transmitted before obtaining the patient's authorization
Remind patients when they do not adhere to the guidelines; if patients repeatedly do not adhere to guidelines, it is acceptable to terminate e-mail communication		
Appropriate messages		
Establish the types of transactions that will be handled via e-mail (prescription-refill requests, appointment scheduling, laboratory/ test results); messages should be short and concise	Provide instructions for when and how to convert to office visits and telephone calls if e-mail is not functioning effectively or if a situation is urgent	Physicians should provide proper notification of e-mail's inherent limitations before the e-mail communication begins or during the first electronic encounter just as one would check on the privacy and safety of a fax or telephone call; if patients initiate e-mail communication, the physician's initial response should include information regarding e-mail limitations and request his or her consent to continue the e-mail conversation
Inappropriate messages		
Messages that require an urgent response, as well as those that address sensitive subject matters (HIV, mental health, etc) are not permitted over e-mail; in addition, avoid anger, sarcasm, or harsh criticism		In e-mail communications, physicians should hold themselves to the same ethical and professional responsibilities as during other encounters

Communications Guidelines	Medicolegal and Administrative Guidelines	Ethics Policy
Sending messages Instruct patients to put the category of transaction in the subject line of the message (prescription-refill request, appointment request, medical advice, etc); request that patients put their name and patient ID number in the body of the e-mail; send a new message to inform patient of completion of request; request that patients use autoreply feature to acknowledge reading clinicians message Provide physician name and contact information at the end of each e-mail; maintain a mailing list of patients, but do not send group mailings in which recipients are visible to each other	Describe security mechanisms in place including password-protected screensaver for desktop workstations at work, hospital, and home; never forward patient-identifiable e-mail to a third party without patient consent; never use patient's e-mail in marketing scheme; do not share professional e-mail accounts with family members; do not use unencrypted wireless communications with patient-identifiable information; check all "to" fields before sending	Physicians should engage in e-mail communication with proper notification of e-mail's inherent limitations; such notice should include information regarding potential breaches of privacy and confidentiality; difficulties in validating the identity of the parties, and delays in responses; physicians should not only rely on disclaimers to convey this information to patients but should provide ongoing medical advice and education to patients in this regard
Storing messages Physicians should retain paper copies of e-mails in medical file (including replies and confirmation of receipt); develop archival and retrieval mechanisms	At least weekly e-mail backup; define time to save paper records	

SOLUTIONS FOR INCREASING PHYSICIAN-PATIENT E-MAIL SECURITY AND VIABILITY

To address many of the logistic and legal issues associated with the use of electronic communication, a number of secure e-mail systems, along with a host of other Web-based services, have been specifically designed to incorporate AMIA/AMA/HIPAA guidelines. Secure Web-based communication services are similar to online banking services or secure e-commerce Web browsers used to purchase goods and services online.[37] They use server-based messaging, firewalls, encryption, and other advanced methods for user authentication. User identification and password authentication for patients, providers, and staff protect patient privacy and account access. These tools verify the authenticity of an individual's identity and ensure that no one besides a doctor and relevant staff have access to specific e-mail. Because these systems are Web-based, they can be accessed from work or school without fear of privacy being compromised by third parties. In addition, time-out features are built in to reduce the chance of accidental viewing by an unauthorized individual in the event that a computer monitor is left unattended.

The following are profiles of 2 companies that provide these services: Medem, a company founded by the AMA and based in San Francisco, California, and RelayHealth Corporation, a privately held company based in Emeryville, California.

Medem

Medem (www.medem.com), supported by several professional organizations including the AMA and the American Academy of Pediatrics, offers a basic, no-frills approach to secure electronic communication. Physicians are provided with a practice Web site that provides patients with information about office location, available hours, and accepted insurance plans. In addition, patients can use the service to schedule office appointments, request renewals of prescriptions, and leave brief messages. In addition, there are structured templates that allow the patient to complete a personal health record (PHR). A new feature, using branching logic, allows patients to describe symptoms before coming in for an acute care visit. It also allows patients to have an online medical consultation with their provider, if desired. Providers have the option of charging a fee for these services, which the system can collect via credit card payment. In terms of health education, providers may direct patients to a library of fact sheets prepared by professional organizations or customize their own educational materials and provide Web links.

In addition to its modest cost and clean architecture, Medem allows youth as young as 12 years to register of their own volition to access the system. According to Jason Best, Vice President of Marketing, Medem recognizes that certain states allow minors to receive confidential services. Therefore, the

Medem system allows "[p]hysicians to practice medicine as they see fit and to interact with their clients based on the various parameters that impact them."

RelayHealth

RelayHealth (www.relayhealth.com) also offers a secure approach to electronic communication between patients and providers, albeit with more features. In addition to the basic items outlined above, patient messages can be triaged to different members of the office staff for appointment and referral requests, queries about billing and insurance, and concerns about medical issues and laboratory results. Structured templates are available to assist the staff to generate quick responses. A broadcast feature allows the provider to send general messages to all patients in the practice or to just a select group. The system will alert the provider in the event that any e-mail remains unopened after a period of time, and the provider has the option of following up, as necessary. In addition, an electronic prescription (e-prescription) service allows providers to e-mail initial or renewed prescriptions to a patient's local pharmacy and puts RelayHealth in compliance with an Institute of Medicine recommendation that by 2010 all providers use e-prescriptions to reduce medication errors.[38]

In terms of clinical services, consumers can complete an intake form that will then be used to create a PHR. The PHR can be modified and updated during clinical encounters. Finally, for minor, nonurgent conditions, patients can arrange for an online Web consultation with their health provider, as described above. Health-education materials, developed by a private company, are available on a variety of topics. Providers can attach these to their e-mail queries. They can also direct patients to Web links for additional information.

Although RelayHealth offers more services (at a higher cost) than Medem, one of the major drawbacks is its minimum age requirement of 18 years. RelayHealth claims that this policy is based on their legal responsibility to ensure that people who sign on to their account are legally recognized by all states to enter into a binding contract to abide by the various rules of the site—a requirement that, in some states, would not apply to people below the age of 18. As a result of our queries and provision of information detailing state guidelines that allow minors to receive a selected menu of services without parental notification, the company is currently discussing a possible policy change: "RelayHealth is researching the possibility of extending its secure Web site services to youth as well as to the adults it now serves in certain states. Just as now—all communications would continue to be done and remain within the secure confines of the RelayHealth website" (Giovanni Colella, MD, President, RelayHealth, written communication, 2007). At present, however, it is not possible for minors to have truly confidential e-mail communication with their physician through this system, because they would be required to share an e-mail account with a parent or family member, thus potentially jeopardizing their privacy.

Although still in need of further development, both of these examples represent a significant upgrade from conventional systems. A comparison of the 2 systems is detailed in Table 2. Relevant issues for adolescents and parents are addressed below.

Specific Issues for Adolescents and Parents

Health Education and Counseling

Secure e-mail systems would seem to be particularly appealing for adolescents in that they present a mechanism for easily accessing providers for routine issues such as requests for appointments or refills of medications. In addition, they also provide the opportunity to "gather one's thoughts" and ask questions electronically. In addition, secure e-mail allows adolescents to maintain contact with a trusted resource even when they are away at camp, vacation, boarding school, or college.[3]

For clinicians who provide services to adolescents, e-mail offers flexibility in the provision of information and health education. As noted previously, patients and families want advice and counseling. However, time is at a premium during most traditional encounters. In addition, patients and families may selectively attend to information presented or misinterpret or forget offered advice.[39] In addition to succinctly summarizing advice and listing instructions in an e-mail, providers may direct patients to view articles in patient-education libraries within secure e-mail systems. However, care must be exercised in selecting and using articles. Currently, the systems are geared primarily for adults. Consequently, materials are "text heavy" and contain few graphics. Providers have the flexibility, however, of populating the library with other resources of their own choosing, thus giving the provider full responsibility for the content. E-mails can also be a useful vehicle for directing adolescents and parents to relevant Web sites for additional reinforcement and guidance, called Web-based information prescriptions or WebIP.[40] Follow-up e-mails may be needed to encourage Web visits. In 1 study, families that received e-mail reminders were found to be more likely (77%) to visit prescribed Web sites than those who were not reminded (53%), which is suggestive of the utility of this approach.[41]

In addition to providing health information, e-mail reminders can assist in increasing adherence to chronic medication regimens. For example, 81% of women on birth control pills miss at least 1 pill per month, and up to 51% miss ≥ 3 pills per cycle.[42] Fox et al,[43] in a study of 40 new oral contraceptive pill users who were receiving daily e-mail reminders, found that 50% reported missing no pills over a 3-month cycle, and 20% missed only 1 in each cycle. Sixty-four percent expressed the desire to continue to receive reminders at the completion of the study.

Secure e-mail may also assist providers in communicating with and providing better support for parents. Parents who are new to the practice may be able to

Table 2
Comparison of secure e-mail systems

Function	RelayHealth	Medem
Cost	Depends on level of service; basic package is $22.50, but additional features cost more; total package (patient messaging, e-prescriptions, colleague messaging) is $112.50/mo or $1350 per physician per year	$395.00/y per physician
Administrative		
HIPAA-ready	Yes; uses secure servers, multiple firewalls, and 128-bit SSL encryption; user ID and passwords are required for both patient and physician access	Yes; uses secure servers, multiple firewalls, and 128-bit SSL encryption; user ID and passwords are required for both patient and physician access
Physician able to list specialty as adolescent medicine	No	Yes
Appointment scheduling	Yes	Yes
Prescription renewals	Yes; patients can request prescription renewals, and provider has the option of using an e-prescription service to electronically send prescription to a pharmacy of the patient's choice	Yes; patient can request prescription renewal; E-script service will be available in late 2007
Workflow and triage capacity	Yes; advanced workflow support allows customization of message-routing rules, distinct roles with proxy right assignment options, support for triage and group coverage models	No; doctors or their staff designees can answer patient e-mails, but there is no triage capability
Structured message format	Yes; clinically structured, branched interviews generate concise, structured messages for clinicians; providers can use structured templates to respond or can use free text	No; patients and providers use free text to communicate

Function	RelayHealth	Medem
Fees and copay collection services	Yes; there are no fees to patients for routine administrative functions, but providers have the option of charging for online consultations; patient credit cards are billed; fees may be reimbursed by some insurance companies	Yes; there are no fees to patients for routine administrative functions, but providers have the option of charging for online consultations; patient credit cards are billed; fees may be reimbursed by some insurance companies
Secure electronic referrals	Yes; secure messaging allows doctors to communicate and refer easily and efficiently within network	No
Clinical		
Clinical review process	Yes; Web-Visit allows patients to consult with physicians; providers can tailor their responses to patient-initiated Web visits with the assistance of medically reviewed, guidelines-based content and attach relevant educational materials	Yes; online-consultation service allows patients to communicate with a physician easily and efficiently; as new modules are added, physicians will be able to get a much broader landscape of adolescent patient background than on a standard office form; also provides a health-risk assessment
Laboratory and test results	Yes; via structured template	Yes; provider enters results as free text in message
Personal health record	Yes, but not specific to adolescents	Yes, but not specific to adolescents
Acute care previsit	No	Yes
Message reminders	Yes	Yes
Features relevant to adolescents		
Online registration for adolescents	No; this feature may be added in late 2007	Yes; minimum age for online registration is 12 y; because laws regarding minors vary by state, Medem leaves decisions about online patient-consultation requirements to individual providers
Educational literature designed for adolescents	No; most literature is directed to parents of younger children	Yes; written by the AAP for both adolescents and parents
Ability to attach customized literature	Yes	Yes

complete surveys (such as the AMA's Guideline for Adolescent Preventive Services parent questionnaire, which solicits areas of concern from parents about their child's health and behavior) before the initial visit. Subsequently, parents can use this medium to bring other concerns before or after the visit and to obtain clarity and reinforcement for any recommendations that were given during the visit. Providers may find the "broadcast" feature in secure e-mail systems helpful to remind parents to bring teens in for flu shots or to schedule annual physicals before the mad dash to complete forms for camp and college in the spring. They can also provide a mechanism for broadly disseminating information about changes in practice policies or insurance plan coverage. In addition, the potential exists to provide parents with education through practice-developed newsletters or links to previously developed resources and materials. For example, the practice can send out information to parents of preadolescent and adolescent girls to alert them of the availability of the new human papillomavirus vaccine and attach a fact sheet that addresses frequently asked questions about the vaccine and the office policies regarding administration and payment.

Clinical Consultations

The ability of secure e-mail applications to provide a mechanism for brief, nonurgent clinical consultations also presents a potential advantage, as long as clear protocols are outlined and followed. For example, a 16-year-old adolescent girl with frequency, urgency, and dysuria may play "phone-tag" for hours, or even days, with her provider's office before getting through to explain her symptoms and receive instructions. By contrast, with secure e-mail, she can fill out an online consultation flow sheet that then can be e-mailed to her provider. After review, the provider may have the option of requiring the patient to come in for an office visit (especially if fever or back pain is present) or, in the absence of systemic signs, may presumptively send an e-prescription to her local pharmacy to begin treatment, along with providing her with a fact sheet about urinary tract infections that details their etiology, management, and prevention. Subsequently, an office visit can be scheduled at a convenient time later in the week to check for resolution of the problem and/or the need to consider other possibilities (if sexually active) such as a chlamydia infection (see Table 3 for more examples).

Special Issues

1. Text messaging: Text messaging has become more common than e-mail among young people in communications with their peers.[6] However, because text messaging occurs over a nonsecure, unencrypted platform, if physicians receive text messages from patients requesting information or advice, they should instruct them to use their secure e-mail system or call the office.
2. Registration: Although some systems allow adolescents to sign up inde-

Table 3
Examples of added value of secure e-mail systems

Content Area	Standard Service Options	Alternative Options Using Secure E-mail
Administrative		
New patient, Mrs Murphy calls the office to schedule an appointment; the next available date is in 2 wk.	At the appointment, she and her son, John, complete registration, family history, and patient history information in waiting room.	She is invited to sign up for secure e-mail, over which she can complete previsit demographic registration, insurance, family medical history, and personal health record. She may choose to relate specific concerns regarding John via the e-mail message before the visit, including his declining grades, moodiness, and unkempt appearance. She is concerned about the possibility of alcohol and drugs playing a role. The provider then has an opportunity to review family history, which shows several family members who have battled with alcoholism, as well as other specific concerns before the visit and may be more focused and armed with helpful resources.
Minor clinical		
Janice Torres, an 18-y-old college student, develops symptoms of a urinary tract infection on a Sunday. Her doctor's office is closed.	Call on Sunday and try to get answering service to reach covering provider; or	Complete Webconsult. The provider reviews the Webconsult and PHR, sees she has no previous history of urinary tract infections and has no allergies.
	Go to the emergency department; or	Contact patient on telephone to clarify info and arrange for evaluation and treatment; or
	Hope symptoms go away with drinking extra fluids; or	Send e-mail message requesting patient to come in to the office in the morning; or

Content Area	Standard Service Options	Alternative Options Using Secure E-mail
	Wait to call Monday; the office may return call while she is in class; she can call back between classes, but provider may be with patients.	Send patient an education guide on urinary tract infections and an e-prescription to pharmacy for Pyridium for comfort until she can come in on Monday; or Send e-prescription into pharmacy for Pyridium and an antibiotic and arrange to see patient for follow-up later in the week to document clearance, assess need for contraception, and sexually transmitted infection screen, and reinforce preventive-education recommendations.
Recurring conditions Ricky Smith, a 17-y-old, presents with intermittent, episodic, temporal headaches; his initial history was somewhat vague and his physical examination unremarkable	Asked to complete headache diary for 2 wk and return for follow-up.	Asked to e-mail reports of any symptoms on a daily basis.
	Loses or forgets headache diary sheet. Returns in 2 wk with incomplete data.	Provider schedules e-mail "prompts" twice a week. Returns in 2 wk: 4 e-mails have been seen showing a pattern of late-afternoon headache, throbbing in nature (5/10), and no associated symptoms; contributing factors include erratic diet and stress related to relationship with girlfriend. Provider focuses discussion on contributing factors and engages patient in dialogue about possible resolution.

Content Area	Standard Service Options	Alternative Options Using Secure E-mail
Confidential question		
Jamie Callender comes in with her mother for evaluation of a rash that is subsequently diagnosed as shingles; she is counseled about the condition and given a prescription; and arrangements are made for follow-up in 1 wk	Jamie seems to have another concern but does not broach it, particularly with her mom in the room.	After her visit, Jamie sends an e-mail indicating that she would like to talk confidentially about contraception at her next visit. Nothing has happened "yet," but she wants to be prepared.
		The provider sends her a note back applauding her courage and honesty and attaches self-care information on contraception, Plan B, and sexually transmitted infections. The provider also directs her to Web sites for more information (www.teenhealthfx.com or www.sexetc.org).
		At her next visit, the provider schedules additional time to allow for extended confidential counseling about sexual decision-making and review of contraceptive methods.
Clarifying information		
Victoria Mallory had unprotected sex yesterday. She goes to her health care provider the next day to get a prescription for Plan B and the NuvaRing.	When she is at the drugstore, she is told to take 1 pill 12 h apart. She thought her provider told her to take both pills at once. In addition, in her anxiety, she misplaced the instructions from the office and is not quite sure when she should insert the NuvaRing. She tries calling the office but gets the answering service. Not wanting to "bother" the doctor after hours, she figures she will call again in the morning.	When Victoria gets home, she logs onto her secure e-mail account and, before she even begins to compose a query, she finds she has a message from the doctor's office waiting for her. It is a standard message that is sent to all patients who receive Plan B, acknowledging how difficult it is to remember a lot of information under stressful circumstances. The message goes on to review how the medication works and how it is administered. In addition, it reviews the procedure for "quick-starting" contraceptive methods, and encourages her to e-mail or call with additional questions or concerns.
		An e-mail appointment reminder is sent to her 1 wk and again 2 d before her next visit.

pendently, others do not. In reviewing standard office policies with parents regarding confidentiality, a sidebar discussion should be held regarding e-mail communication.[37] If parents feel comfortable with this, they can register themselves and their adolescents. Similarly, discussions should be held with adolescents about the importance of e-mail communication etiquette (ie, not sharing passwords, not leaving a computer screen unattended, logging off after use, etc).

3. Inappropriate use: Finally, although the guidelines outlined above are clear regarding the appropriate use of e-mail for electronic communication, there have been situations in which patients have not used the system as it was intended. For example, in a study of adults, although most of the patient-generated queries were appropriate, 21% dealt with urgent issues such as suicidal ideation.[2] Given the nature of adolescents and their health concerns, providers may reasonably expect to receive queries that should not be handled via electronic communication. Patients should be encouraged to use other forms of communication to address these concerns. If these types of inappropriate communications continue, providers have the right to terminate the privilege altogether.

CONCLUSIONS

Given adolescents' familiarity with and predilection toward electronic forms of communication, providers should consider incorporating secure e-mail systems into their office practices. Although still "rough around the edges," these systems have untapped potential to improve office efficiency and enhance communication between providers, adolescents, and parents.

ACKNOWLEDGMENT

This work was supported by Centers for Disease Control and Prevention grant U48-DP000030.

REFERENCES

1. Hobbs J, Wald J, Jangannath Y, et al. Opportunities to enhance patient and physician e-mail contact. *Int J Med Inform*. 2003;70:1–9
2. Houston TK, Sands DZ, Jenckes MW, Ford DE. Experiences of patients who were early adopters of electronic communication with their physician: satisfaction, benefits, and concerns. *Am J Manag Care*. 2004;10:601–608
3. Cohall A, Cohall R. Why you should consider "messaging" with your patients and parents by e-mail and the Web. *Contemp Pediatr*. 2004;21:76–88
4. Fox S, Madden M. Pew Internet & American Life Project: generations online. Available at: www.pewinternet.org/pdfs/PIP_Generations_Memo.pdf. Accessed May 11, 2007
5. Gold R, Atkinson N. Communicating health: priorities and strategies for progress. Available at: http://odphp.osophs.dhhs.gov/projects/healthcomm/objective1.htm. Accessed May 11, 2007
6. Lenhart A, Madden M, Hitlin P. Pew Internet & American Life Project: teens and technology—youth are leading the transition to a fully wired and mobile nation. Available at: www.pewinternet.org/pdfs/PIP_Teens_Tech_July2005web.pdf. Accessed May 11, 2007

7. Centers for Disease Control and Prevention. Annual rate of visits per person to physician offices by patient age group: United States, 2003. *MMWR Morb Mortal Wkly Rep.* 2005;54(48):1238. Available at: www.cdc.gov/mmwr/preview/mmwrhtml/mm5448r9.htm

8. Fairbrother G, Scheinmann R, Osthimer B, et al. Factors that influence adolescent reports of counseling by physicians on risky behavior. *J Adolesc Health.* 2005;37:467–476

9. Schor EL; American Academy of Pediatrics, Task Force on the Family. Family pediatrics: report of the Task Force on the Family. *Pediatrics.* 2003;111(6 pt 2):1541–1571

10. Ferris TG, Saglam D, Stafford RS, et al. Changes in the daily practice of primary care for children. *Arch Pediatr Adolesc Med.* 1998;152:227–233

11. Kane B, Sands D. Guidelines for the clinical use of e-mail with patients. *J Am Med Inform Assoc.* 1998;5:104–111

12. Bauchner H, Adams W, Burstin H. You've got mail: issues in communicating with patients and their families by e-mail. *Pediatrics.* 2002;109:954–956

13. Harris Interactive. Patient/Physician online communication: many patients want it, would pay for it, and it would influence their choice of doctors and health plans. *Health Care Rep.* 2002;2:1–3

14. Harris Interactive. Few patients use or have access to online services for communicating with their doctors, but most would like to. Available at: www.harrisinteractive.com/news/allnews-bydate.asp?NewsID=1096. Accessed May 11, 2007

15. Allen K, Raine L. Pew Internet & American Life Project: parents online. Available at: www.pewinternet.org/pdfs/PIP_Parents_Report.pdf. Accessed May 11, 2007

16. Anand SG, Feldman MJ, Geller DS, Bisbee A, Bauchner H. A content analysis of e-mail communication between primary care providers and parents. *Pediatrics.* 2005;115:1283–1288

17. Baraff LJ, Wall SP, Lee TJ, Guzy J. Use of the internet and e-mail for medical advice and information by parents of a university pediatric faculty practice. *Clin Pediatr (Phila).* 2003; 42:557–560

18. Goldman RD, MacPherson A. Internet health information use and e-mail access by parents attending a paediatric emergency department. *Emerg Med J.* 2006;23:345–348

19. Cohall A, Cohall RM, Ellis JA, et al. More than heights and weights: what parents of urban adolescents want from health care providers. *J Adolesc Health.* 2004;34:258–261

20. Hutchinson JW, Stafford EM. Changing parental opinions about teen privacy through education. *Pediatrics.* 2005;116:966–971

21. Kaiser Family Foundation. Generation Rx.com: how young people use the internet for health information. Available at: www.kff.org/entmedia/upload/Toplines.pdf. Accessed May 11, 2007

22. Valaitis, Ruta R. Computers and the Internet: tools for youth empowerment. *J Med Internet Res.* 2005;7(5). Available at: www.jmir.org/2005/5/e51

23. American Medical Association. Guidelines for physician-patient electronic communications. Available at: http://ama-assn.org/ama/pub/category/print/2386.html. Accessed May 11, 2007

24. Kassirer J. Patients, physicians, and the Internet. *Health Aff (Millwood).* 2000;19:115–123

25. Manhattan Research, LLC. *Taking the Pulse 3.0: Physicians and Emerging Information Technologies.* New York, NY: Manhattan Research, LLC; 2003

26. Kleiner KD, Akers R, Burke BL, Werner EJ. Parent and physician attitudes regarding electronic communication in pediatric practices. *Pediatrics.* 2002;109:740–744

27. American Academy of Pediatrics, Division of Health Policy Research. *Periodic Survey of Fellows 51: Use of Computers and Other Technology.* Elk Grove Village, IL: American Academy of Pediatrics; 2003

28. Patt MR, Henckes MW, Sands DZ, Ford DF. Doctors who are using e-mail with their patients: a qualitative exploration. *J Med Internet Res.* 2003;5:e9. Available at: www.jmir.org/2003/2/e9

29. White CB, Moyer CA, Stern DT, Katz SJ. A content analysis of e-mail communication between patients and their providers: patients get the message. *J Am Med Inform Assoc.* 2004;11:260–267

30. Sands DZ. Help for physicians contemplating use of e-mail with patients. *J Am Med Inform Assoc.* 2004;11:268–269

31. Kind T, Huang ZJ, Pomerantz KL. Internet and computer access and use for health information in an underserved community. *Ambul Pediatr.* 2005;5:117–121

32. Institute of Medicine. *Crossing the Quality Chasm: A New Health System for the 21st Century.* Washington, DC: Institute of Medicine; 2001

33. Brooks RG, Menachemi N. Physicians' use of e-mail with patients: factors influencing electronic communication and adherence to best practices. *J Med Internet Res.* 2006;8:e2. Available at: www.jmir.org/2006/1/e2

34. Weiss N. E-mail consultation: clinical, financial, legal, and ethical implications. *Surg Neurol.* 2004;61:455–459

35. HIPAA Security Rule: Health Insurance Reform—Security Standards. *Fed Regist.* 2003;68: 8334–8381

36. Gerstle RS; American Academy of Pediatrics, Task Force on Medical Informatics. E-mail communication between pediatricians and their patients. *Pediatrics.* 2004;114:317–321

37. Delbanco T, Sands DZ. Electrons in flight: e-mail between doctors and patients. *N Engl J Med.* 2004;350:1705–1708

38. Institute of Medicine. Report brief: preventing medication errors. Available at: www.iom.edu/Object.File/Master/35/943/medication%20errors%20new.pdf. Accessed May 11, 2007

39. Tang PC, Newcomb C. Informing patients: a guide for providing patient health information. *J Am Med Inform Assoc.* 1998;5:563–570

40. D'Alessandro DM, Kreiter CD, Kinzer SL, Peterson MW. A randomized controlled trial of an information prescription for pediatric patient education on the Internet. *Arch Pediatr Adolesc Med.* 2004;158:857–862

41. Ritterband LM, Borowitz S, Cox DJ, et al. Using the Internet to provide information prescriptions. *Pediatrics.* 2005;116(5). Available at: www.pediatrics.org/cgi/content/full/116/5/e643

42. Potter L, Oakley D, de Leon-Wong E, Canamar R. Measuring compliance among oral contraceptive users. *Fam Plann Perspect.* 1996;28:154–158

43. Fox MC, Creinin MD, Murthy AS, Harwood B, Reid LM. Feasibility study of the use of a daily electronic mail reminder to improve oral contraceptive compliance. *Contraception.* 2003;68: 365–371

Adolesc Med 18 (2007) 293–304

Internet Surveys With Adolescents: Promising Methods and Methodologic Challenges

Erika Sutter, MPH*, Jonathan D. Klein, MD, MPH

Division of Adolescent Medicine, University of Rochester, 601 Elmwood Avenue, Box 690, Rochester, NY 14642, USA

The most profound change of the information age is the growth of the Internet. For an ever-increasing proportion of the population, cyberspace and the World Wide Web offer immediate connectivity and expanded social-networking opportunities across time and space without traditional geographic limitations. These changes have implications for health care and for health-services and clinical research. Web-based surveys have the potential to provide research data quickly and efficiently,[1,2] reach more potential respondents, provide greater access to "hidden" population groups, allow rapid, convenient input by respondents, and reduce bias in respondents' replies to questions about sensitive topics.[1] Although the use of Web-based surveys in health and behavioral research is expanding, limitations of using this methodology also exist. Sampling issues, especially self-selection and how to provide representative samples using Web-based panels, are important factors in Web-based surveys. Although 73% of US adults and 87% of US youth aged 12 to 17 use the Internet, demographic and geographic disparities in Internet access still exist.[3,4] Web-based survey data can be weighted to reflect population demographics in ways that are similar to methods used in national household and telephone surveys.[2,5] However, whether this bias resulting from self-selection into survey samples can be effectively adjusted for has been central to the debate over online-survey validity.[2] Text-based Web surveys also require greater literacy skills and exclude both those without Internet access and those whose manual dexterity or visual acuity does not allow computer-based responses. Confidentiality, identity, and other ethical issues also must be taken into consideration in online-survey development. Here we review current

---

*Corresponding author.

E-mail address: erika_sutter@urmc.rochester.edu (E. Sutter).

All data referenced in this article are available from public sources. The authors do not endorse any single vendor or sample source for Web-based surveys.

Financial Disclosure: Dr Klein collaborates with Harris Interactive survey methods scientists on studies using Harris Poll Online and other Internet surveys. He does not receive compensation from Harris Interactive; however, he has access to proprietary data on sample and propensity weighting and has agreed to maintain the confidentiality of those materials. Ms Sutter has indicated she has no financial relationships relevant to this article to disclose.

literature and some of the benefits and challenges of Web-based survey research with adolescent and young adult populations.

WEB-BASED SURVEY RESEARCH: AVAILABILITY OF SURVEY SOFTWARE TOOLS

Web-based surveys have been used with adolescent populations in various settings. In thinking about these surveys, it is useful to differentiate between surveys of known groups of respondents using the Internet as a mode of presenting questions and those surveys that use unique aspects of the Internet in developing their sample frame. In both cases, computer-assisted survey presentation allows items to be visually formatted and allows skip patterns, rotation of response categories, and other means of targeting respondents, resulting in both less respondent burden and more complete exploration of specific answers or issues.

Computer-based surveys that use Internet software to reach a known population are increasingly common, especially with the rise of simple, low-cost, menu-driven software that allows development of questionnaire items and simple analyses without technical programming expertise. In general, these surveys involve either written or e-mailed invitations that respondents answer from any Internet-compatible computer at their convenience. Some programming packages also allow for customization of skip patterns (eg, skipping unnecessary questions and allowing targeted follow-up queries), which results in greater efficiency.

For example, the American College Health Association offers colleges and universities the option to administer the National College Health Assessment, a health-risk–behavior survey for college students, via paper and pencil or on the Web. If the Web-based option is chosen, students are invited to participate via an e-mail message that contains a link to complete and submit the survey online. A reminder e-mail is sent to nonresponders; data transmission is encrypted, and firewall securities are in place.[6] In 1999, an experimental study was conducted by using the National College Health Risk Behavior Survey[7] to compare a mailed, self-administered survey with a Web-based survey version.[8] The Web-based sample was contacted via e-mail and received a cover letter with a link to the survey Web site. The authors found that response rates as well as demographic characteristics of both the mail and Web samples were similar and that offering the Web-based survey version was a feasible option for a university population.[8]

Many computer software packages are available for designing Web-based surveys. A recent Google search for "survey software" returned 172 million results, and "Web-based survey software" returned 71 500 Web sites and numerous software companies. Alternatively called Web-survey, Internet-survey, or online-survey software, these products help the user to design and administer surveys, track nonrespondents, and even analyze results.[9] These sites allow researchers to collect data from hundreds up to thousands of respondents at minimal or no cost. However, researchers should be cautious in purchasing these packages. Careful consideration of whether and how basic formatting and screen appearance can be controlled, whether list-based responses can be rotated (to avoid acquiescence or "top-box" bias), whether data are easily exportable to analytic programs, comparability to other sources or to historical data, and other methodologic and technical issues should be considered before selecting a Web-based method. It is likely that these methods will continue to spread. For example, the Centers for Disease Control and Prevention (CDC) plans to migrate its Youth Risk Behavior Surveillance System to computer-administered formats by 2009 or 2011 (L. Kann, PhD, CDC, Division of Adolescent and School Health, verbal communication, 2006).

SAMPLING ISSUES IN WEB-BASED SURVEY RESEARCH

Surveys that use unique aspects of the Internet in developing their sample frame as well as in survey administration are encountered less frequently in medical or public health literature. Nonetheless, Web-based survey research methods have grown substantially in recent years, primarily reported in sociology and market-research fields. These surveys share some of the same methodologic issues as computer or Web-based survey studies that use small, defined populations or known samples. However, almost all Internet-sampled surveys are provided by a handful of market-research firms, most of which have customized and sophisticated approaches to questionnaire and response design standards. Although these surveys can incur costs substantially greater than that from the do-it-yourself software packages, access to the population of respondents is a significant benefit without which many studies could not be performed. However, Internet-based sampling requires careful assessment of sample and response bias and validity and reliability issues.

Web surveys can be administered in different ways: (1) a survey may be sent via e-mail, and the respondent would send the completed survey back via e-mail; (2) a survey invitation may be sent via e-mail with a direction or an embedded link to a Web site that contains the actual survey; or (3) respondents may be invited to participate in a survey via advertisements or recruitment from off-line and/or online sources (eg, ads posted on a popular Web site, postal letters with a Web site address, etc).[2] In the first 2 cases, respondents are invited on the basis of their e-mail address, which raises obvious questions about how well individuals can be sampled from e-mail addresses. In the third case, samples may be recruited with varying degrees of certainty depending on the nature of the lists or other sources from which subjects are invited. However, self-selection into survey samples has been criticized, and whether this type of bias can be adjusted or controlled for successfully has been central to the debate over their validity.[2] In each of these scenarios, invitations can contain unique links or may allow either a single or multiple responses from individual IP (Internet protocol) addresses. Although it might seem appropriate to limit responses to 1 per IP address, IP addresses can be shared by multiple devices or may be assigned as needed by a Web server; thus, an IP address may belong to a Web host (ie, an academic setting or cable television company server) rather than to an individual end user.

Response rates may be difficult to calculate for a Web-based survey (eg, if the survey is administered on a public Web site on which any site visitor potentially has the opportunity to take the survey but may choose not to). E-mail invitations, on the other hand, are usually drawn from a specific group or panel of preidentified potential respondents; thus, a response rate is calculated more easily. Web-survey response rates vary widely and depend on sampling procedures, incentives, and the characteristics of the population being surveyed.[9,10] However, 1 meta-analysis of response rates in electronic surveys from both published and unpublished research found that response representativeness was more important than response rates in the Web studies analyzed.[11]

Web-based surveys have increasingly been seen as useful in developing samples that are representative of the population, especially as completion rates from traditional telephone-survey methods have dropped.[12–14] Telephone surveillance has become challenging because of the increasing use of cell phones, call-screening/blocking devices, and number portability, all of which adversely affect survey-completion rates and sample frames.[10,13,15–18] As cell-phone usage continues to grow, telephone samples become individual rather than household based, and the geographic nature of number assignment becomes blurred.[17] Although some studies have shown that nonresponse bias is minimal even for noncoverage of households without landline telephones,[14,19] this issue should continue to be studied as telephone technology is adapted.

Although household samples (such as those used in the US Census and in the CDC's National Health Interview Survey) remain the gold standard of representativeness, household interviews are both time and labor intensive, and recent literature suggests that nonresponse rates are also increasing with this method.[20] The face-to-face nature of household interviews may influence respondents' answers to questions about sensitive topics such as sexual behavior or illicit drug use. However, computer-assisted questionnaires have been used during household surveys to minimize social-desirability bias and obtain more accurate self-report on sensitive topics such as these.[21–23]

Krosnick and Chang[24] reported on a study that compared completion rates and data quality across different strategies for online samples, including (1) comparison of Knowledge Network's identification of a household frame, obtaining consent, placing Internet-access devices connected to television sets, and inviting participation in surveys, and (2) the Harris Interactive Internet panel (the Harris Poll Online). The Harris Poll Online has >6 million US members who have

Table 1
Key considerations in Internet-survey research

Benefits	Ability to obtain data quickly and efficiently
	Potential to reach large numbers of respondents
	Web-based surveys allow rapid, convenient input by respondents
	Extensive availability of online-survey software helps users design and administer surveys, track nonrespondents, and analyze results
	Electronic questionnaires may lessen social-desirability bias and eliminate interviewer effects
	Survey data can be weighted to reflect population demographics
	Web surveys are able to accommodate unique design features (such as audio or visual content)
Challenges	Although Americans' access to the Internet is expanding, demographic and geographic disparities still exist
	Careful assessment of sample bias (eg, self-selection) and response bias is needed
	Response rates may be difficult to calculate in certain samples
	Representativeness of the sample should be considered
	Literature regarding validity and reliability of Web-based samples is limited; more research is needed
	Online surveys may require greater literacy skills and may exclude those with physical limitations who are unable to use a computer
	Confidentiality and other ethical issues may present new challenges to researchers

volunteered to participate in surveys on topics from consumer products to health behaviors and conditions and uses propensity weighting to adjust responses for the likelihood of being online and of responding to a particular survey's E-mail invitation.[2] Although much has been made of the relative advantages of either sampling method by corporate stakeholders, both methods lose high and comparable proportions of respondents (albeit at different points in their enrollment and sampling processes with respect to an individual survey query), and both have been challenged with regard to representativeness of their results. However, a number of studies have indicated substantial comparability for both approaches.[24–28]

Currently, 73% of US adults and 87% of US 12- to 17-year-olds use the Internet[3,4]; however, demographic and geographic disparities still exist. In early 2006, the Pew Internet & American Life project found that adults aged 18 to 49 were much more likely to use the Internet than those over the age of 65; similarly, 63% of rural households had access to the Internet at home, compared with 75% of urban and 75% of suburban households.[3] In addition, in 2003, there was ~1 wireless telephone for every 2 persons in the United States, and 46.6% of all US telephones were wireless.[19] In 2005, 8.4% of all US adults were estimated to live in households without a landline telephone. Of these, 1.7% had no telephone service at all, for whom the respondents with no telephone service for part of the year are reasonably representative. In contrast, 6.7% of all US adults and 13.6%

of those under the age of 25 are in cell-phone–only households.[19] Thus, some researchers have suggested that mixed-mode approaches will be needed to accurately represent the entire population.[10,15,25,29]

National household and telephone surveys require weighed analyses to adjust for cluster-sampling designs, and most also adjust for undercoverage and underresponse of certain sections of the population (most notably those who are poorer and those who are members of some ethnic minority groups).[17,19] Online-survey data can similarly be weighted to reflect population demographics.[2,24] For example, Bethell et al[30] obtained a representative sample of the US population in a 2003 study of health care system quality by using a large panel sample and additional weighting procedures. Similarly, we have shown that national self-reported prevalence estimates of current cigarette use are comparable between a large online panel sample compared with estimates from several national telephone and household-interview surveys.[31]

CHALLENGES OF INTERNET SURVEYS

There are a variety of methodologic threats to using Internet surveys. Many of these issues are also true of different traditional methods; however, some are unique to the online-survey mode, and others are exacerbated by use of the computer for simultaneous response and data input.

Some Web-based survey-mode effects are similar to those of mailed self-administered paper-and-pencil surveys. These effects include the ability of the respondent to review or change previous answers or to skip ahead or back to other questions. In contrast to some paper-and-pencil surveys, Web surveys allow multitasking while taking the survey, and respondents can start and stop at any time. These effects are difficult to track, although timing for completion of items can be measured by using customized survey programming, and this makes possible quantification of respondent burden and any item-nonresponse effects attributable to subject fatigue. In addition, because Web surveys are generally self-administered, the relative anonymity of electronic questionnaires may lessen social-desirability bias and eliminate interviewer effects.[1,10,32]

Nonresponse and sample issues may also be present in Web surveys (eg, if respondents do not receive an e-mail invitation because they infrequently access their e-mail account).[10] Similarly, respondents may have multiple e-mail accounts, either in or external to the sample frame. Multiple responses from individuals may or may not be able to be tracked, although some opinion-research companies have tried to estimate the magnitude of repeat or frequent responders and have successfully adjusted for the effects of these "professional" or "hyperactive respondents" on data.[33] Web-based data collection eliminates interviewer effects, which may help to minimize item nonresponse within the survey itself. Survey designers have the ability to insert prompts that call attention to items that the respondent may have left blank (providing a "second chance" or requiring that the subject enter a response) and, therefore, decreasing the likelihood that a survey will contain missing data.[34]

Relatively few studies to date have examined whether survey respondents provide different information depending on the mode of delivery; although this may depend on the samples used and on the nature of the questions being asked, a recent study showed no evidence of a mode effect with Web-based questionnaires.[35]

As with other survey modes, choices of item format for online surveys also impact survey responses. Item format has been shown to significantly affect attitude and prevalence estimates for non–health behaviors, with formats dependent on greater respondent attention resulting in lower estimates (eg, a multiple-response item list will provide lower estimates than a series of yes/no responses).[36,37]

MIXED-MODE APPROACHES

In recent years, mixed-mode approaches for data collection have been explored as a means of providing a more-comprehensive representation of population groups.[8,10,17] Combining Web-based survey methods with traditional methods such as household or telephone interviewing may decrease costs and alleviate challenges associated with decreasing response rates and inadequate telephone coverage.[10] Although some studies have shown that demographic and other characteristics of Web and mail or telephone sample groups were not significantly different,[8] others have found that demographics and even some health behaviors and attitudes of Web respondents varied considerably from those of telephone or mail respondents.[2,16,38] Galesic et al[10] reported that mixed-mode data collection with a Web-based component may be most useful when a sufficient number of respondents are willing and able to respond on the Web, when differences in data quality across modes are minimal, and when there is a benefit to offering the Web-based mode, such as higher response rates or reduced costs. However, Link and Kresnow[17] point out that telephone-survey methods will continue to be conducted in the foreseeable future, although additional research on alternative modes of data collection is necessary. Although the literature base is growing,[15,39–42] more methodologic research on mixed-mode approaches of data collection is likely needed to obtain conclusive evidence on which approaches are best suited to different population groups and survey topics.

UNIQUE LIMITATIONS AND STRENGTHS OF INTERNET SURVEYS

Web-based survey methods have been found to be both time and cost efficient compared with telephone random-digit-dial methods.[2] Many Web-based surveys have reduced costs compared with other survey methods.[13] Automated data collection and data entry take place as respondents complete the survey online, thus reducing the need for hiring staff for this purpose. Researchers also save money by not needing to print and mail surveys, train interviewers to administer the survey, or provide space for survey administration and storage.[1] In a recent Web-based study of adolescents' use of complementary and alternative medicine, we were able to obtain a weighted, nationally representative sample of 1300 respondents from Harris Interactive's youth panel over a 1-week field period.[43] Thus, Web-based surveys have the potential to reach large numbers of respondents in a short period of time and may be a useful component of future studies of the US population.[31] However, Harris Interactive respondents are initially recruited via e-mail, popular Web sites, mail, and other methods, and both panel membership and participation factors may influence estimates in other, unknown ways.[31]

Web surveys are unique in that numerous design features can be added to surveys on the basis of the researcher's needs. For example, some survey software or interfaces allow for item randomization or response randomization for part or all of a survey. Audio or video clips or other visual components may be added to expand items or improve comprehension of or explain survey content.[10,13] Online surveys also allow for easy branching, or automatically skipping items that do not apply to a respondent on the basis of their previous responses.[9] Drop-down menus, radio buttons, and other data-entry options specific to Web-based surveys help to facilitate data entry as well as minimize response error.[1]

One of the challenges in online sampling, whether data are weighted for demographics, propensity, or both, is that participant identity is based on self-representation. Depending on the circumstances, an online participant's self-representation may not reflect a respondent's true, real-world identity. As mentioned above, Internet users often have >1 e-mail address, and bad addresses and nondelivery may be difficult to account for, making the meaning of nonresponse less clear; quality measures for panel performance have only recently been developed.[33] Variation in Internet access, including the speed and type of connections, may also influence participants' responses and possibly their likelihood of completing surveys.[44]

Computer-based survey methods also may underrepresent low-literacy populations and people with disabilities. Text-based Web surveys generally require greater literacy skills than do other methods, and keyboard or mouse use may exclude potential participants' whose manual dexterity or visual acuity does not allow computer-based responses. Although adaptations to ensure equal access to the Internet and development of assistive technologies for these populations are possible, they are rarely used in practice.[1]

VALIDITY AND RELIABILITY OF INTERNET SURVEYS WITH ADOLESCENTS

An extensive review of the validity and reliability of Web-based surveys is beyond the scope of this review; however, several groups are examining data quality and various presentation and item-format effects on responses and estimates from online surveys.[24,31,36,41,45–47] In addition, Bethell et al[30] found that health care quality-measurement surveys designed for administration by mail and telephone maintained psychometric reliability and concurrent validity across demographic and other subgroups when administered online. Although most of these studies were in adult populations, we have demonstrated test-retest reliability of reproductive health surveillance comparing online and telephone methods.[48,49]

CONFIDENTIALITY AND OTHER ETHICAL ISSUES

Identification of IP addresses and/or e-mail addresses may be of concern to respondents depending on the sensitivity of a survey's content.[1] The identification of a sample by e-mail only may also present new challenges to both researchers and institutional review boards.[50] In some cases, affirmative identification may be appropriate; however, allowing panel members to respond with self-representation of eligibility may also be needed to ensure that respondents' privacy is adequately protected. These issues become magnified when subjects are cognitively mature minors. Federal guidelines for involvement of those under age 18 in research are open to interpretation based on minimal risk and lack of feasibility of obtaining identity confirmation without greater potential for harm. In contrast, the International Code of Marketing and Social Research Practice, which was jointly drafted by the International Chamber of Commerce and European Society for Opinion and Market Research, a Europe-based international society whose members include the American Association of Public Opinion Research, allows involvement of adolescents in studies.[51] The federal Children's Online Privacy Protection Act of 1998 requires that commercial Web sites obtain verifiable parental consent before collecting personal information from a child under the age of 13 and specifies that the Federal Trade Commission would view failure to obtain such consent an unfair and deceptive trade practice. In addition, companies are required to maintain reasonable procedures "to protect the confidentiality, security, and integrity of personal information collected from children."[52] Some online-survey firms also explicitly state more restrictive age and privacy standards.[53]

Although without interviewer effects, online surveys make it more difficult to identify respondents' needs for support or crisis services (eg, if a respondent experiences distress as a result of the research) than in face-to-face or telephone surveys.[1] Although a resource list could be provided on the survey screen, respondents and the researcher are likely to be asynchronous, in separate locations, and local resources may not be provided on such a list. This is an issue that researchers should anticipate and address as survey projects are designed.

CONCLUSIONS

Web-based surveys and the use of Web-panel samples have great potential for survey research. Many methodologic questions remain to be explored. Nonetheless, these methods can accurately represent many adolescent and young-adult populations and will be an increasingly relevant part of how we learn about the attitudes and behaviors of youth in our society.

ACKNOWLEDGMENT

We thank Randall K. Thomas, Director of Internet Research at Harris Interactive, for review and comment on an early version of this manuscript.

REFERENCES

1. Rhodes SD, Bowie DA, Hergenrather KC. Collecting behavioural data using the World Wide Web: considerations for researchers. *J Epidemiol Community Health.* 2003;57:68–73
2. Schonlau M, Zapert K, Simon LP, et al. A comparison between responses from a propensity-weighted Web survey and an identical RDD survey. *Soc Sci Comput Rev.* 2003;21:1–11
3. Pew Internet & American Life Project. Demographics of Internet users. Available at: www.pewinternet.org/trends/User_Demo_4.26.06.htm. Accessed December 21, 2006
4. Lenhart A, Madden M, Hitlin P; Pew Internet & American Life Project. Teens and technology: youth are leading the transition to a fully wired and mobile nation. Available at: www.pewinternet.org/pdfs/PIP_Teens_Tech_July2005web.pdf. Accessed December 30, 2006
5. Pew Internet & American Life Project. Internet: the mainstreaming of online life. Available at: www.pewinternet.org/pdfs/Internet_Status_2005.pdf. Accessed December 30, 2006
6. American College Health Association. National College Health Assessment. Available at: www.acha-ncha.org/index.html. Accessed December 21, 2006
7. National Center for Chronic Disease Prevention and Health Promotion, Division of Adolescent and School Health. Youth Risk Behavior Surveillance: National College Health Risk Behavior Survey—United States, 1995. *MMWR CDC Surveill Summ.* 1997;46(6):1–56
8. Pealer LN, Weiler RM, Pigg RM Jr, Miller D, Dorman SM. The feasibility of a Web-based surveillance system to college health risk behavior data from college students. *Health Educ Behav.* 2001;28:547–559
9. Solomon DJ. Conducting Web-based surveys. *Pract Assess Res Eval.* 2001;7(19). Available at: http://pareonline.net/getvn.asp?v=7&n=19
10. Galesic M, Tourangeau R, Couper MP. Complementing random-digit-dial telephone surveys with other approaches to collecting sensitive data. *Am J Prev Med.* 2006;31:437–443
11. Cook C, Heath F, Thompson RL. A meta-analysis of response rates in Web- or Internet-based surveys. *Educ Psychol Meas.* 2000;60:821–836
12. Curtin R, Presser S, Singer E. Changes in telephone survey nonresponse over the past quarter century. *Public Opin Q.* 2005;69:87–98
13. Tourangeau R. Survey research and societal change. *Annu Rev Psychol.* 2004;55:775–801
14. Keeter S, Kennedy C, Dimock M, Best J, Craighill P. Gauging the impact of growing nonresponse on estimates from a national RDD telephone survey. *Public Opin Q.* 2006;70:759–779
15. Mokdad AH, Stroup DF, Giles WH; Behavioral Risk Factor Surveillance Team. Public health surveillance for behavioral risk factors in a changing environment: recommendations from the Behavioral Risk Factor Surveillance Team. *MMWR Recomm Rep.* 2003;52(RR-9):1–12

16. Link MW, Mokdad AH. Alternative modes for health surveillance surveys: an experiment with Web, mail, and telephone. *Epidemiology.* 2005;16:701–704
17. Link MW, Kresnow M. The future of random-digit-dial surveys for injury prevention and violence research. *Am J Prev Med.* 2006;31:444–450
18. Kristal AR, White E, Davis JR, et al. Effects of enhanced calling efforts on response rates, estimates of health behavior, and costs in a telephone health survey using random-digit dialing. *Public Health Rep.* 1993;108:372–379
19. Blumberg SJ, Luke JV, Cynamon ML. Telephone coverage and health survey estimates: evaluating the need for concern about wireless substitution. *Am J Public Health.* 2006;96:926–931
20. Groves RM. Nonresponse rates and nonresponse bias in household surveys. *Public Opin Q.* 2006;70:646–675
21. Sieving RE, Beuhring T, Resnick MD, et al. Development of adolescent self-report measures from the National Longitudinal Study of Adolescent Health. *J Adolesc Health.* 2001;28:73–81
22. Turner CF, Ku L, Rogers SM, Lingberg LD, Pleck JH, Sonenstein FL. Adolescent sexual behavior, drug use, and violence: increased reporting with computer survey technology. *Science.* 1998;280:867–873
23. Holbrook AL, Green MC, Krosnick JA. Telephone versus face-to-face interviewing of national probability samples with long questionnaires: comparisons of respondent satisficing and social desirability response bias. *Public Opin Q.* 2003;67:79–125
24. Krosnick JA, Chang LC. A comparison of the random digit dialing telephone survey methodology with Internet survey methodology as implemented by Knowledge Networks and Harris Interactive. Presented at: the 56th Annual Conference of the American Association for Public Opinion Research; May 18, 2001; Montreal, Quebec, Canada
25. Chang L, Krosnick JA. National surveys via RDD telephone interviewing vs. the Internet: comparing sample representativeness and response quality. Presented at: the 56th Annual Conference of the American Association for Public Opinion Research; May 18, 2001; Montreal, Quebec, Canada
26. Krosnick JA, Nie N, Rivers D. Comparing the results of probability and non-probability sample surveys. Presented at: the American Association for Public Opinion Research Conference; May 14, 2005; Miami Beach, FL
27. Taylor H, Bremer J, Overmeyer C, Siegel JW, Terhanian G. The record of Internet-based opinion polls in predicting the results of 72 races in the November 2000 US elections. *Int J Market Res.* 2001;43:127–135
28. Thomas RK, Krane D, Taylor H, Terhanian G. Attitude measurement in phone and online surveys: can different modes and samples yield similar results? Presented at: the European Association of Methodology (EAM) Society for Multivariate Analysis in Behavioral Sciences (SMABS) Conference; July 5, 2006; Budapest, Hungary
29. Schonlau M, Asch BJ, Du C. Web surveys as part of a mixed-mode strategy for populations that cannot be contacted by e-mail. *Soc Sci Comput Rev.* 2003;21:218–222
30. Bethell C, Fiorillo J, Lansky D, Hendryx M, Knickman J. Online consumer surveys as a methodology for assessing the quality of the United States health care system. *J Med Internet Res.* 2004;6:e2. Available at: www.jmir.org/2004/1/e2
31. Klein JD, Thomas RK, Sutter E. Self-reported smoking in online surveys: prevalence estimate validity and item format effects. *Med Care.* 2007;45:691–695
32. Bowling A. Mode of questionnaire administration can have serious effects on data quality. *J Public Health (Oxf).* 2005;27:281–291
33. Smith R, Brown HH. Panel and data quality: comparing metrics and assessing claims. Presented at: the European Society for Opinion and Market Research Panel Research Conference; November 28, 2006; Barcelona, Spain
34. Fricker S, Galesic M, Tourangeau R, Yan T. An experimental comparison of Web and telephone surveys. *Public Opin Q.* 2005;69:370–392
35. Denscombe M. Web-based questionnaires and the mode effect: an evaluation based on completion rates and data contents of near-identical questionnaires delivered in different modes. *Soc Sci Comput Rev.* 2006;24:246–254

36. Thomas RK, Klein JD. Merely incidental: effects of response format on self-reported behavior. *J Off Stat.* 2006;22:221–244

37. Smythe JD, Dillman DA, Christian LM, Stern MJ. Comparing check-all and forced-choice question formats in Web surveys. *Public Opin Q.* 2006;70:66–77

38. Link MW, Mokdad AH. Effects of survey mode on self-reports of adult alcohol consumption: a comparison of mail, Web and telephone approaches. *J Stud Alcohol.* 2005;66:239–245

39. de Leeuw E. To mix or not to mix data collection modes in surveys. *J Off Stat.* 2005;21:233–255

40. Link MW, Mokdad A. Can Web and mail survey modes improve participation in an RDD-based national health surveillance? *J Off Stat.* 2006;22:293–312

41. Christian LM, Dillman DA, Smyth JD. The effects of mode and format on answers to scalar questions in telephone and Web surveys. Presented at: the 2nd International Conference on Telephone Survey Methodology; January 12, 2006; Miami, FL

42. Dillman DA, Phelps G, Tortora RD, Swift K, Kohrell J, Berck J. Response rate and measurement differences in mixed mode surveys: using mail, telephone, interactive voice response, and the Internet. Available at: http://survey.sesrc.wsu.edu/dillman/papers/Mixed%20Mode%20ppr%20_with%20Gallup_%20POQ.pdf. Accessed January 8, 2007

43. Wilson KM, Klein JD, Sesselberg TS, et al. Use of complementary medicine and dietary supplements among U.S. adolescents. *J Adolesc Health.* 2006;38:385–394

44. Dillman DA. *Mail and Internet Surveys: The Tailored Design Method.* New York, NY: Wiley & Sons, Inc; 2000

45. Klein JD, Thomas RK, Sutter E. Validity of self-reported cardiovascular disease risk factors in online samples. Presented at: the American Public Health Association Annual Meeting; November 6, 2006; Boston, MA

46. Ritter P, Lorig K, Lauren D, Matthews K. Internet versus mailed questionnaires: a randomized comparison. *J Med Internet Res.* 2004;6:e29. Available at: www.jmir.org/2004/6/e29

47. Dillman DA, Smyth JD, Christian LM, Stern MJ. Multiple answer questions in self-administered surveys: the use of check-all-that-apply and forced-choice question formats. Presented at: the American Statistical Association Annual Meeting; August 5, 2003; San Francisco, CA

48. Klein JD, Havens CG. Internet survey methods: reliability and mode effects. Presented at: the 11th World Congress on Internet and Medicine-MedNet Conference; October 17, 2006; Toronto, Ontario, Canada

49. Klein JD, Havens CG. Adolescents' and young adults' social networks in cyberspace. Presented at: the 11th World Congress on Internet and Medicine-MedNet Conference; October 17, 2006 Toronto, Ontario, Canada

50. Eysenbach G, Wyatt J. Using the Internet for surveys and health research. *J Med Internet Res.* 2002;4:e13. Available at: www.jmir.org/2004/4/e13

51. European Society for Opinion and Market Research. ESOMAR world research codes & guidelines: interviewing children and young people Available at: www.esomar.org/uploads/pdf/ps_cg_interviewingchildren.pdf. Accessed January 3, 2007

52. Federal Trade Commission. Children's Online Privacy Protection Act of 1998: Title XIII—children's online privacy protection. Available at: www.ftc.gov/ogc/coppa1.htm. Accessed January 8, 2007

53. Harris Interactive. Privacy policy. Available at: www.harrisinteractive.com/about/privacy.asp. Accessed January 8, 2007

Adolesc Med 18 (2007) 305–324

Has the Internet Changed Everything or Nothing? Thoughts on Examining and Using Emerging Technologies in Adolescent Health Research

Dina L. G. Borzekowski, EdD*

Department of Health, Behavior, and Society, Johns Hopkins Bloomberg School of Public Health, 624 North Broadway, #745, Baltimore, MD 21205, USA

In this article, 2 ways of thinking about emerging technology and adolescent health research are examined. Given the limited (albeit growing) number of published studies, this discussion is presented through a case-study approach. To illustrate a given relationship or method, recent studies are offered as examples. After discussing the purpose and findings, a study's strengths and weaknesses are highlighted, not to praise or disparage a researcher's work but, rather, to critique the research methodology. The article concludes with a description of common concerns in adolescent research and suggestions for ways that we can advance the field of emerging technologies and adolescent health research.

THE USE AND IMPACT OF EMERGING TECHNOLOGIES AND TODAY'S ADOLESCENTS

A Wired World

Today's teenagers live in a wired world; new technologic devices fill adolescents' everyday environment and even their personal wardrobe. The average American child lives in a media-rich household; 73% of children have ≥ 3 television sets, 97% have a VCR, DVR, or DVD player, 86% have a computer, and 83% have a video-game system.[1] Among 8- to 18-year-olds, two thirds have a television set in their bedroom, and approximately one third of teenagers (11- to 18-years-olds) have a computer in their bedroom.[1] Practically all US teenagers, 87% of those aged 12 to 17 years, regularly use the Internet, and 51% report

---

*Corresponding author.
E-mail address: dborzeko@jhsph.edu (D. L. G. Borzekowski).

that they go online daily.[2] Nearly half (45%) of US teenagers carry their own cell phone, and more than half have iPods or MP3 players.[3]

Access to new technology is not limited to the United States. Among French adolescents, most (85%) report ownership of a cell phone.[4] In Finland, cell-phone ownership is practically universal (99%) among adolescents.[5] In Asia, adolescent Internet use is widespread; research on urban youth from Seoul, South Korea, Singapore, and Taipei, Taiwan, found that 91% had home access to the Internet.[6] Emerging technologies are also popular in developing countries. In Ghana's capital of Accra, two thirds (66%) of in-school adolescents and slightly more than half (54%) of the out-of-school adolescents have used the Internet.[7] In rural Uganda, 45% of students indicated that they were Internet users; averages from the 5 sampled secondary schools ranged from 11% to 91% of the students using the Internet.[8]

Media multitasking is common, with adolescents using ≥ 2 media at a given time. Simultaneous media use can involve watching television, listening to music, using the Internet, and communicating with friends. Reports from US youth indicate that the typical 8- to 18-year-old is exposed to an average of 8½ hours of media content per day, although he or she is just spending 6 hours 21 minutes using media.[1] When asked about television viewing, half the sampled teenagers reported that some or most of the time they are also listening to music, reading, or using a computer.[1] Recent research with American 18- to 24-year-olds suggests that Internet use comprises 23% of a young person's media time, followed by watching television (22%) and listening to MP3 players (19%).[3] Another recent nationwide study found that 74% and 83% of the time that US adolescents e-mail and instant message, respectively, they are also using other media.[9]

Across ages, people turn to new technology for similar purposes. The majority of users turn to the Internet and cell phones to better communicate with friends and family. The latest and growing trend is to turn to the Internet for social network-ing, especially among older teenagers. Social-networking Web sites (ie, MySpace, Facebook, Xanga) are sites on which users can create their own page and connect with others. A recent study of US teenagers found that 70% of girls and 57% of boys aged 15 to 17 have created their own online profiles.[10] Daily use is common; 26% of social-networking–site users visit profile pages once a day, and 22% visit several times per day.[10]

In addition, the Internet is also a great resource for various types of information; surveys consistently report that users go online for entertainment, product, and health information.[2] Although concern has been raised about the quality of online health information,[11] the nature of technologies, in contrast to in-person inter-actions with health providers, allows ease of access in an anonymous and nonpunitive way.[12] Sensitive information is often searched for online, especially among young people. With sexual information being the most popular topic, similar rates for looking up health information among online adolescents have been observed in North America and Africa.[7,13,14]

Technology's Impact

Since the introduction of electronic media and technology, researchers have been interested in whether and how its use is associated with different health outcomes. Extensive literature exists that spans across different disciplines, showing that adolescents' use of various media (print, radio, television, video games, and computers) is associated with everything from obesity to violence, academic performance, and social interactions.[15–18]

Since the late 1990s, studies have been released on how the use of emerging technologies is associated with different health outcomes. The HomeNet Project, which followed 10- to 19-year-old users of the Internet from 1995 to 1997, found that more boys than girls were using the Internet.[19] As availability grows, however, this gender difference seems to be breaking down; however, boys and girls still do different things while they are online. Both use the Internet for communication and information purposes, but boys are significantly more likely to play computer and online games.[19]

"Widely publicized but preliminary," there was an impression that Internet use would have a negative influence on the social development of its young users.[20] Not based on solid research, reports were disseminated that the typical Internet user would be behind a closed door, typing on a keyboard and meeting up with online strangers, many of whom might alter and try on different identities. Additional concern was raised that too much time online would lead children to lack interpersonal skills.[21]

Now that the Internet is more widespread, we are seeing more sound studies that consider how use of these technologies relates and predicts various outcomes. As an example, Gross[20] returned to the earlier propositions to reexamine if frequent Internet use would be associated with depression and social isolation. Participants offered data on their Internet use and their household media environment. More than 200 middle and high school students provided diary data on the context and characteristics of their online experiences. Participants also completed measures that assessed levels of loneliness, social anxiety, and depression.

Gross[20] found no significant gender differences with regard to overall usage; however, there was a small group, mostly of boys, who were avid game players and spent a greater time online. For the study participants, the majority of online time was devoted to private communication. Reportedly, interactions with strangers were infrequent; for boys and girls, communication was with friends from school using the instant-message function. Time on the Internet was not associated with the adolescents' psychosocial adjustment, including daily measures of isolation and well-being. Lastly, Gross found no significant evidence that the Internet is an environment that promotes anonymous identity play and exploration. Of those who reported that they had pretended to not be themselves online, the characteristic they most frequently altered was their age.

A recent study with >4000 Finnish adolescents offers some interesting data to consider on the health of online users. Lajunen et al[5] examined the association of overweight status with computer and cell-phone use and ownership among a population-based sample of adolescent twins. First considering ownership from 2001 to 2005, the researchers found that among surveyed 17-year-olds, the proportion of those with household computers increased from 82% to 92%, and home Internet access increased from 61% to 81%. Over the same data-collection period, cell-phone ownership increased from 88% to 99%.

The researchers found that adolescents with a household computer were at higher risk of being overweight compared with those without a household computer; however, weekly computer hours nor Internet access was associated with weight status.[5] Increased cell-phone use, as measured with monthly cell-phone bills, was related to higher BMI. Findings were adjusted for a host of variables including gender, engagement in physical activity and exercise, and parents' education and occupation.[5]

Media Messages and Adolescents

Media-effects studies will often use time as a critical predictor, although there is consensus that it is content that truly matters. Researchers are trying to understand what the messages are that adolescents are exposed to through emerging technologies. Studies explore what general and specific populations of youth are seeing and hearing through new media.

The Internet offers countless and wide-ranging Web sites on every imaginable topic. As noted earlier, for young people in the United States and abroad, an important topic often accessed is health. The most common subjects considered are gender, diet, and exercise; however, many young people use new technology to address their own mental health and special needs.[7,12,13] Through the Internet, a young person can find information about sensitive topics without the embarrassment or geographical or temporal difficulties involved in communicating with an in-person health provider.

In several studies, Borzekowski and Rickert[13] examined if general groups of adolescents sought health information online. In a study of 412 New York high school students, the researchers found that among those who had gone online for personal health information, 42% had looked up information on sexual activity, contraception, and pregnancy. An equal percentage had tried to find information on fitness and exercise. Approximately 15% had looked up mental health issues.

Considering online health information, students reported high levels of worth, trustworthiness, use, and relevance regardless of their gender, ethnicity, or mother's education.

With a carefully drawn sample of 778 in-school and out-of-school teenagers who lived in Ghana's capital city of Accra, Borzekowski et al[7] discovered similar findings regarding adolescents' online health seeking. Among Internet users, 45% said that they had looked up information about sexually transmitted diseases (including HIV/AIDS), and 33% had used the Internet to find information about sexual activities. One third (33%) reported that they had gone online for diet and nutrition information. Ghanaian youth described online health information as useful, easy to read, trustworthy, and relevant.[7]

Albeit limited in their generalizability, fascinating research exists on several different vulnerable groups and online information. Boyer et al[22,23] examined a small sample of 12 adolescent drug users, all of whom had reportedly used the Internet to find information on psychoactive drugs. An often-cited Web site was www.erowid.org. All study participants (9 boys, 3 girls) stated that they had learned novel information and had altered their drug knowledge and behaviors by drawing on this online information. Information influenced most of the individuals' drug use, but interestingly, 8 of the participants detailed how Internet information and Web sites had taught them ways to minimize risks.[22]

In another study of how vulnerable adolescents turn to the Internet for health messages, researchers surveyed 182 individuals (76 patients, 106 parents) who attended an eating disorder clinic and their use of pro–eating disorder and prorecovery Web sites.[24] Half (51%) of the patients reported that they had visited either site type; 36% said they had gone to pro–eating disorder Web sites, 41% had gone to prorecovery sites, and 25% had gone to both site types. Practically all (96%) pro–eating disorder Web-site users reported that they had learned new methods of weight loss or purging online, and 69% indicated that they had tried the new method.[24]

RESEARCH APPROACHES AND EMERGING TECHNOLOGY

Not only adolescents but also many adolescent health researchers are turning to emerging technologies. To conduct and better understand adolescent health, researchers consider and use new media in their exploration and practice. Not surprisingly, familiar and traditional designs are common and I describe below how researchers are using observational, cross-sectional, and experimental designs. I also describe the ways in which emerging technologies can facilitate data collection and other research tasks.

Observational Research

To investigate adolescent health, researchers often go where the adolescents are and observe their behaviors. One way of understanding behaviors with new media is to monitor the existing information environment to which young media users are exposed. Researchers can monitor the number and nature of electronic health messages that an individual encounters through content-analysis methodology; a content analysis involves the systematic sampling of a given media and the subsequent coding of specific and explicit references to a particular topic.

Recently, the content-analysis methodology was used to better understand the messages presented on self-injury Web sites.[25] Self-injury refers to when an individual inflicts harm to his or her body in a way that is neither socially sanctioned nor for the purpose of committing suicide. These behaviors are done to regulate emotion and are cries for attention.[26] Self-injurers perform cutting, which is the intentional carving or scraping of the skin but also the burning, ripping, bruising, or breaking of skin and bones. Prevalence rates of nonsuicidal self-injurious behaviors among adolescents are estimated to be between 13% and 23%.[26]

Whitlock et al[25] investigated 10 Web sites for 2 months and examined 3219 posts on self-injury message boards. These boards maintained low and medium moderations, meaning that submitted messages were not strictly reviewed before being posted, and there was a strong potential for potentially damaging messages to be on the board (ie, postings that explained how to self-injure). Dominant themes of the posted messages included supportive statements for others (28%), discussion of events that trigger self-injury (19%), and concealment issues (9%). Of all the posts, 7% involved comments about formal help-seeking from physical and mental health providers. Although 19% of the help-seeking comments presented negative attitudes, 44% were positive. The remaining 37% referred to therapies or medications.[25]

Another recent content analysis explored the messages offered through pro–eating disorder Web sites, which are sites that offer advice and encouragement to those who want to maintain their eating disorders.[27] Elements of the extended parallel processing model[28] were considered and used as a theoretical framework to code the content that appeared on proanorexia and probulimia Web sites. This behavior change and communication model was used to analyze which Web sites might offer more effective messages. An initial Google search provided a list of 106 Web sites; however, only messages from 19 sites were included in the analysis. Some 1600 distinct messages were coded into the theoretical categories of severity (3%), susceptibility (1%), response efficacy (48%), self-efficacy (2%), and nonrelevance (46%).[27] Lapinski[27] suggested that these sites are not as harmful as they could be, because the response-efficacy messages were not coupled with self-efficacy messages. In fact, the reverse seems to have been true:

only an exclusive and unique group of people could achieve the recommended responses involved in maintaining eating disorders.

These 2 content analyses represent examples of how researchers observe the existing online environment.[25,27] If one were to use this methodology in future work, it would be advisable to attend to 3 aspects of the design: sampling, unit of analysis, and reliability.

Sampling for Internet content analyses needs to be done with a great level of rigor, more so than has been observed in recently published studies. For example, in the Whitlock et al self-injury analysis,[25] an initial search uncovered 406 sites; however, only 10 were selected for the analysis. The researchers purposely chose message boards with low and medium moderation. Similarly, the Lapinski study[27] only examined one fifth of the sites revealed in their Google search. The initial output of Google was screened for inclusion of a home page, menu, list of links, list of tips, regular activity, and presentation in English.[27] To make valid and generalizable claims about the available messages presented on certain Web sites, a systematic and carefully planned population must be determined. Using Google is a fine strategy, because it is and has been the most popular search engine for years. Too many inclusion and exclusion criteria of output, however, can bias a content analysis' findings. I would recommend that samples for online content analysis be randomly drawn from a more inclusive population.

A second and important consideration in performing a content analysis is establishing an unambiguous unit of analysis. For example, if one were to perform a content analysis by analyzing smoking messages on television, one might identify the unit of analysis to be character or scene. Results would then be presented as the percentage of characters or scenes that contain references to smoking. In the Whitlock et al study,[25] the units were message board and then individual posts. In the Lapinski study,[27] the unit was Web sites. In examining online messages, researchers should declare a clear unit of analysis. With a clear unit, researchers may describe the percentage of sites, pages, or messages that refer to a topic at hand.

A third consideration in content analyses is the reliable and clear definition of the attribute in question. Independently, different coders ought to come up with the same number of references if they were to examine the same media. Imagine a Web site that offers text, audio, and video messages about smoking. To come up with an accurate count of the messages, previous decisions need to be made as to whether inhaling and exhaling smoke is the only acceptable version of smoking or if holding a lit cigarette or open package is also regarded as smoking. As was done in the study of self-injury message boards, the coding team decided and defined in advance what would characterize the various and potential themes.[25]

Cross-sectional Research

If one wants to understand how 2 variables relate (eg, use of emerging media and an adolescent health issue), a cross-sectional research design might be in order. Adolescent health researchers can use this design to collect a large amount of data from their participants. Researchers pose questions to their study participants through either surveys or interviews. Collected data can be analyzed, and relationships can be determined in a straightforward manner, resulting in useful and relevant information in a timely and less-expensive way.

Surveys

Researchers have turned to schools, health centers, and even street corners to collect information from adolescents on their use of electronic media and related outcomes.[29] In one study, a sample of Korean senior high schools students was drawn, and researchers examined, through a cross-sectional design, the characteristics of those who used the Internet to excess.[30] Representing schools from different economic districts, 328 students completed a questionnaire package that included several different batteries assessing media use, psychological symptoms, and personality traits. The students were categorized into 4 groups: nonusers (18%), minimal users (47%), moderate users (30%), and excessive users (5%). Using analyses of variance with posthoc comparisons, the researchers observed that excessive users had significantly higher scores than minimal users on several symptom subscales (ie, somatization, obsessive/compulsive, interpersonal sensitivity, depression, anxiety, hostility, phobic anxiety, and psychoticism), suggesting higher levels of pathology for those who reported excessive Internet use.[30] Interestingly, the nonusers also reported significantly greater levels of pathology for 7 of the 9 subscales, which suggested a certain degree of psychiatric symptomatology among those who did not have exposure to the Internet. When considering personality trait scores, the excessive users were not significantly different from the youth in the other Internet-user groups.[30]

Interviews

Another way to collect data on the use and impact of emerging technologies is to use the long-standing method of interviewing. Several publications on current trends regarding adolescents and new media derive from the first and the second Youth Internet Safety Survey data sets. These surveys used telephone interviews that drew from a national panel of Internet users between the ages of 10 and 17 years and their parents.[31,32] From participating households, researchers spoke with youth and their caregiver for 30 and 10 minutes, respectively. In the first study, the researchers found that among youth who used the Internet regularly ($N = 1501$), 25% were exposed to unwanted online sexual material in the last year.[31] Exposure was associated with older age, higher household income, and more Internet use. Interestingly, children whose parents monitored their Internet use more were also more likely to have exposure to online sexual material.[31] In the second survey, the telephone interviews of 1500 10- to 17-year-olds revealed that 42% were exposed to online sexual material, and two thirds of those youth said the exposure was unwanted.[32] Among those who reported that they had exposure to wanted materials, there was a greater likelihood that they had been harassed online and had received unwanted online sexual solicitations.[32]

Although the cross-sectional design can offer information on the presence of significant relationships, it precludes claims about causal inferences.[5] As described earlier, the work of Lajunen et al[5] showed that computer ownership and cell-phone use is related to BMI among adolescents; however, this design did not allow the researchers to determine the directionality of the observed relationship. Similarly, in the Yang et al work,[30] the data showed significant relationships, but it was not possible to discern whether the observed psychological symptoms preceded or resulted from the excessive Internet use. The Internet may form an outlet for those with poor social relationships, few friends, dissatisfaction with physical appearance, and poor coping skills.[33] Possibly, a preoccupation with and reliance on electronic technology to facilitate relationships may lead to problems such as depression, anxiety, and low self-esteem.[34]

Cross-sectional research also cannot explain if other potential or unobserved confounders are influencing the relationships between emerging technologies and health status. In reference to the studies on exposure to online sexual material, it is very possible that there is something about the individual that predicts that they would not only see these materials but also be the victims of harassment and solicitation.[32]

As with the earlier content-analysis method, a critical aspect of cross-sectional research is one's sampling approach. Using surveys or interviews may produce large samples, but the question that often remains is how generalizable one's sample will be. Consider the aforementioned Youth Internet Safety surveys. In these studies, ~1500 people participated in the studies; however, this reflected a 45% response rate.[31,32] The authors relied on a random-digit-dial approach to obtain their samples, which can be problematic for several reasons. To begin, there has been an overall decline in willingness to participate in telephone surveys. Poor response rates reflect the do-not-call list, caller ID, and exclusive use of cell phones.[35] In addition, the topic of online pornography is a "charged" one, and it is possible that the topic altered one's willingness to participate.[32] Even once people agreed to participate, it is likely that some subjects were too embarrassed to admit seeking out or wanting to see online sexual material.[32] Questions about validity often arise when data collection uses self-report and disclosure of sensitive material.

Experimental Research

Several recent studies examined the impact of messages delivered via new media through experimental designs. Researchers collected baseline data, randomly assigned participants into online intervention versus control groups, and then obtained additional data at a later time. Such an approach is considered the gold standard for determining the impact or effect of exposure or a given variable. In most experimental research of this type, an intervention is created, and participants are encouraged to turn to the intervention materials through their cell phone or computer.

Using a participatory and experimental research design, Woodruff et al[36] investigated whether use of a virtual online world coupled with motivational interviewing by a smoking-cession counselor could reduce adolescent smoking. Adolescent smokers from southern Californian high schools were recruited to join a study to help researchers "learn more about teen smoking." After being surveyed at baseline, 136 participants were randomly assigned to either the invention or control groups. Randomization to condition occurred by school rather than participant to avoid contamination between control and interventions groups and facilitate delivery of the protocols and intervention program.[36]

All participants were reminded via telephone and regular mail to complete their online surveys. In addition, they were paid incremental amounts to complete surveys. A virtual environment was created for intervention-group participants. In the virtual world, which resembled a shopping mall, participants could select an avatar (a 3-dimensional figure), visit different settings within the mall, and have real-time discussions with other participants and smoking-cessation counselors.[36]

Immediately after the 7-week intervention, researchers found significant differences between the adolescents in the intervention and control groups for abstaining from cigarette smoking. This difference was not sustained; participants were nearly identical at the 3-month follow-up assessment. Interestingly, at the 12-month follow-up, intervention participants had significantly more "quit attempts," and more of them described themselves as former smokers at the 12-month follow-up.[36]

Another experimental study examined if and how an Internet-based education program (IEP) could improve the self-management skills of asthmatic children and adolescents.[37] As part of this work, the researchers performed a cost/benefit analysis of using the Internet to deliver the program. This study was conducted in Germany, and 438 asthmatic patients aged 8 to 16 from 36 study centers participated. For several reasons, including severity of illness, urgency of education, and required Internet access, this investigation used a nonrandomized, nonstratified approach of 2 intervention groups. The single control group consisted of patients who would receive the intervention 6 months after the study.[37]

Patients in both of the intervention groups took part in a standardized patient-management program (SPMP) that involved educational sessions in which patients learned skills (ie, use of inhaler devices, classification of medications, awareness and avoidance of triggers) and participated in role-playing exercises. In addition, study participants could self-select into an IEP. The IEP (available at www.asthmax.de) featured educational material, individualized medication plans, quizzes, and interactive adventure-game communication tools to chat and e-mail with patients and providers.[37]

Despite design limitations, Runge et al[37] found interesting and significant findings. Participation in the SPMP, and especially the added IEP, resulted in higher quality-of-life measures, less school absenteeism, fewer asthma-related emergencies, and decreased use of short-acting β agonists. Within 1 year of the study, morbidity cost savings exceeded the intervention costs, especially among the moderately and severely ill patients. The benefit/cost ratio of the SPMP was 0.55; the added IEP significantly improved the ratio to 0.79.[37]

In 2006, Williamson et al[38] reported findings from their randomized, controlled trial. These researchers tested the efficacy of an Internet-based program over a 2-year period with 57 overweight black girls (mean age: 13.2 years) from Louisiana. Participants were randomly assigned into groups. The intervention consisted of access to a Web site that delivered nutrition education and behavior modification for the participating girls and their parents, e-mail communication between the participants and nutrition counselors, and various interactive components (eg, quizzes, lessons, goal-setting exercises). Participants were encouraged to self-monitor and record online their weight, food intake, and physical activity; input data were converted into visual graphs. The control group received similar information to that of the online group; however, this information was delivered through face-to-face interactions and Web sites that promoted healthy lifestyles.[38]

Outcome measures for the study included BMI, body fat, and weight-loss behaviors. In addition, the study examined Web-site use by recording the frequency of log-on sessions to the secured Web sites. Williamson et al found that participants in the intervention group lost significantly more weight and body fat during the first 6 months of this trial, compared with those in the control group. Participants in the intervention group frequently visited the recommended Web sites, and many entered their weight and physical activity during the first year of the study. Although short-term differences were apparent, group differences faded over time; no significant differences were associated with group by the final data collection (at 24 months).[38]

Using Technology in Data Collection

In adolescent health studies, emerging technologies are used to assist implementation and ease research tasks. Researchers may use cell phones and Web sites as novel ways to engage and improve adherence to protocols. In many situations, technology also facilitates the research process and enables otherwise difficult and burdensome tasks.

Researchers can use technology to attract young participants (especially those who are vulnerable and hard to reach) into studies and increase participation. For example, researchers have been examining the feasibility and logistic challenges in improving adherence to behavioral and medical protocols. In a pilot study, 8 adolescent participants were given a new and free cell phone and phone cards and regularly received reminder calls to take their highly active antiretroviral therapy medication for HIV treatment.[39] The 12-week intervention, which involved reminder calls, was found to be practical for the research staff and agreeable to the study participants. During the intervention, practically all the participants adhered to the medications and had lowered viral loads. At postintervention, however, patients returned to their earlier behavioral and medical conditions of nonadherence and high viral loads, respectively.[39]

A finding across several of these studies that tried to attract and engage young people is that for the short-term, technology seems to be having an impact. Youth will use the new media, which seems to influence their health behaviors. After a few weeks, however, the lure weakens. Most of these studies do not show prolonged effects.

One consistent benefit of emerging technology is that it can ease research tasks. In previous years, the audio-supported computer-assisted self-interview (A-CASI) methodology has been introduced and warmly accepted in adolescent health research. This method, in which participants hear questions and then enter responses into a computer, can reduce literacy demands on study participants.[40] Because A-CASI allows for higher levels of privacy over the standard paper-and-pencil or interview approaches, studies that use this method often find higher reports of sensitive or risky behaviors.[41]

A-CASI demands computer resources and often requires researchers to set up school or clinic laboratories in which participants can access the data-collection systems. The use of personal digital assistants (PDAs) improves on the A-CASI methodology, because it further removes barriers for participation. PDAs offer great flexibility, more so than laptop computers, because they are easy to carry, transport, and recharge. In a middle school setting, researchers evaluated the use of an audio-enhanced PDA (APDA) system with 645 students.[42] Unlike paper-and-pencil surveys, students were excited to participate and were respectful of the equipment. The APDA was well liked by 96% of the students, and across those with different reading and language abilities, there was a high level of ease in using the system. Also, the research field staff appreciated the APDA system. It required less effort to carry and set up, no data were lost, and files were immediately available for analysis.[42]

When studies involve emerging technology, researchers can quite likely use innovative systems to monitor aspects of participation. Automatic and electronic records can reliably determine if, when, and how long an individual visits a restricted Web site. For example, in the Runge et al[37] study of an IEP for asthmatic children, the researchers were able to determine from their computer provider that, on average, patients were logged onto the study site for 2 hours per month. They could also know that the most visited sites were the peak flow–protocol section, the chat room, and the adventure game.

CRITICAL RESEARCH ISSUES

Researchers are using traditional and innovative approaches to collect data and understand the relationship between emerging technologies and adolescent health. Certain issues transcend all types of adolescent health research, and I discuss several of these issues here, including effective recruitment and retention of participants, obtaining proper consent, protecting confidentiality of participants, and collecting reliable data.

Recruitment, Participation, and Retention

Throughout health research, recruiting study participants can be challenging, especially when the study topic involves delicate or even illegal topics. Furthermore, research that involves multiple assessments, various tasks, and even slightly complex protocols suffers from poor participation and retention. Although there are exceptions, research that examines or uses new media with young people endures problems in recruiting, engaging, and retaining the samples.

From a medical chart review, Wilson et al[24] identified 698 potential participants and sent out a single mailing to previous and current patients (who were ≥18 years old at the time of the study) at an eating disorder clinic and their parents. Researchers received 182 completed surveys, reflecting response rates of 11% and 15% of patients and parents, respectively. In discussing the response rate and the potential bias of participants, the researchers suggested that the volatile nature of pro–eating disorder Web-site use may have prevented willingness to participate.

Koo and Skinner[43] studied recruitment strategies involved in obtaining adolescent samples for online health research. In a targeted recruitment approach, the researchers invited registered members of a youth health Web site. Describing different incentive amounts ($20 and $30), 3801 e-mails were sent and adolescents were asked to go to a Web site to complete a study. Close to 1700 e-mails were undeliverable. Assuming that the remaining 2109 e-mails were received, it is astounding that just 11 potential subjects visited the study Web site, and only 5 subjects (0.24%) satisfied the recruitment criteria and completed the survey.

More encouraging findings for online recruitment were found by Gordon et al[44] preceding their study of an online smokeless tobacco–cessation program. To evaluate the effectiveness of different strategies, these researchers tried multiple approaches including paid advertisements on Google, referrals from other Web sites, media (print, radio, and television) coverage, paid advertisements in newspapers, and direct mailings to health providers. Approximately 3600 people began the screening process, and eventually 2523 participants enrolled in the study. Approximately half of the participants (51%) had heard of the study through the media coverage, and another 35% came to the study though Google and the other Web sites. Examining the costs involved in recruitment, the researchers estimated the lowest per-participant rate ($6.70) was for using Google and the other Web-site referrals. The media campaigns cost approximately $92 per participant. Advertising in the newspapers had a $115 rate, and the direct mailings cost $597 per participant.[44]

Once individuals are enrolled onto a study, there is often a level of participation that is expected and necessary. To examine the impact of messages delivered via new technologies, participants often have to go online and visit a predetermined Web site.[37,38,45]

In smoking-cessation research that examined the impact of a virtual online world, researchers observed immediate, albeit short-term, results.[36] Although some long-term results were observed, researchers were extremely disappointed with the level of participation among subjects. Despite efforts and ever-increasing subject payment, 19% of the intervention participants never attended any of the virtual world's online sessions. One problem was that the design required a smoking-cessation counselor to be present and monitor the virtual world, which limited the times that participants could access the intervention. Very limited participation was also observed in a study that investigated an online alcohol-misuse–prevention course among college freshman.[46] Of the 310 students in the experimental group, 173 completed the follow-up survey. Approximately half had performed all 5 online units, whereas the other half had performed none of the units.

Retention varies across studies of emerging technology and, as in other types of research, depends on the context and content of the research. A study that examined the impact of online sex education that was given through high schools and colleges in Shanghai, China, managed to follow-up with a remarkable 97% of its 1337 recruited subjects.[47]

Often, interventions that try to improve hard-to-change behaviors are small and have low completion rates; also, these trends are observed in the programs that use emerging technology. In a smoking-cessation study that used both Web-site and cell-phone text messaging, researchers began the study with 46 college-aged participants.[45] By the end of 6 weeks, data from only 29 participants were available. Trying to reduce weight, the Williamson et al[38] study began with 57 overweight black girls. At 24 months, just 40 participants remained in the study. Although these numbers allowed tests of significance, the loss of participants frustrated the researchers, given the tremendous effort involved in creating the program. Interestingly, the researchers suggested that the use of innovative delivery systems may also function as a limitation; this sample of black participants may have preferred a cooperative rather than individualized and computer-driven program.[38]

Consent

It is valuable to examine young people's relationship with emerging technology; however, established safeguards required in other settings should not be abandoned. The Internet can deliver sensitive and even risky messages to young people, and studies on use and impact should involve consent of participants and, in the case of minors, active parental permission. Wilson et al[24] encountered problems when trying to recruit patients with an eating disorder and their parents into their study of pro–eating disorder Web sites. Understandably, parents were concerned that participation in the research might introduce their already vulnerable children to harmful online content.

When research occurs through electronic channels, consent is a more-elusive process. Online research often relies on the participant completing a pop-up consent screen and trusts that the individual has read and understood the study's objectives and potential risks and benefits. Interestingly, many online surveys do not involve active parental consent even when the participants are younger than 18 years. In a study of a teen sexually transmitted disease–prevention Web site (www.iwannaknow.org), a random sample of users were invited to participate, and 42% of the 3489 participants were between the ages of 13 and 17 years. Those who reported that they were <13 years of age were thanked for their interest and returned to the Web site's homepage.[48] Despite (or maybe because of) the inclusion of questions on different risk behaviors (sexual intercourse, drug and alcohol use), these participants were not required to have their parents' consent to participate.

Other online research seems to avoid the consent issue, presumably because it involves virtual ethnography. This is extremely contentious because the online world, although clearly a public space, is considered by many of its users as private. Bypassing or actively circumventing consent is unacceptable when collecting information about young people. For instance, it is objectionable to lurk in and collect data from users of chat rooms, especially if the researcher has not identified himself or herself. In addition, it seems questionable to consider and analyze information on personal social-networking sites, especially among underage participants. It is unlikely that young Web-site users post information in private chat rooms or member-only Web sites with the expectation that researchers will be inspecting their communication.

Anonymity and Confidentiality

Studies that involve emerging technologies may be confidential, but for the most part, they are not truly anonymous. Although the principal investigator may be hard-pressed to find such information, most information technologists and data managers can affirm that practically all electronic messages contain identifiable information. Even data offered to an "anonymous" online survey can be traced back to a unique Internet-protocol address.

Research indicates that users' foremost concern in turning to the Internet for health information involves privacy.[49] Research and interventions must involve strong protection of confidentiality; steps need to be taken to password-protect Web sites and encrypt electronic messages.[50] Despite these measures, adolescents often are a hard-to-protect group. Although advised otherwise, young people will share hardware (ie, cell phones, PDAs) and give out their passwords.

Reliability and Validity

Many studies rely on participant self-report data, and the question often asked is, how reliable are instruments delivered through emerging technology? Initial studies suggested that the psychometrics of online measures resemble those completed through traditional data-collection methods.[51–53]

Researchers examined different administration of the Child Health Questionnaire Child Form by randomly assigning 1071 adolescents into different administration modes. The authors found that those who completed the Internet version compared with the paper mode had fewer missing answers. Psychometric properties, however, were equal between study administrations.[53] With a sample of college students, Fortson et al[52] compared the internal consistency and correlations between measures using Internet and paper formats. Not only were the findings consistent with previous research, but the students' information on traumatic events and psychological symptoms were stable across research sessions and formats.

Parsimonious instruments, delivered through cell phones, PDAs, and/or Web sites, may not be able to capture the qualitative nature of events and behaviors with new media. For example, much of the publicized and highlighted research on online safety relies on a handful of questions asked over the telephone.[35] In research on online safety and harassment, respondents answered ~25 questions that reflected on the most-bothersome event they had encountered. This set of questions was only asked if the participant initially revealed a positive response to 1 of just 2 questions. With worrisome events and sensitive issues, it may be inappropriate to use conventional approaches and limited questions; more open-ended, in-depth approaches should be used.

Especially in research that concerns emerging technology, more-objective measures are possible. Researchers may ask participants to self-report and estimate the number of hours they spend using certain media, but in fact, researchers can obtain and verify reported time with actual bills from cellular-network providers.[5] As an example, Williamson et al[38] were able to assess Web-site use by recording the total number of hits on the overall Web site and number of hits on the personalized pages on which participants monitored their weight and physical activity.

CONCLUSIONS AND RECOMMENDATIONS

Griffiths et al[54] conducted a systematic review of early online interventions, and their findings offered some explanations for why emerging technologies will continue to play a developing and prominent role in adolescent health research. To begin, emerging technology offers an attractive way to deliver health interventions and research methods to young people. This age group has grown up with media multitasking; from communication to education to entertainment to health-seeking, there is little that young people do that does not involve emerging technology. In addition, emerging technology can offer delivery of research or interventions at increased convenience and reduced costs to the research team and participants. New media modes can reach many more people at a time, so the rate per participant is much less than would be otherwise. Rather than an effort that goes out to a general population, the use of technology allows adolescent health researchers to reach narrow groups with targeted approaches. Instead of standardized and unnecessary components, emerging technology can provide sensitive and specific materials. Usual barriers such as geography and time fade as researchers can reach isolated groups, outside of regular school, work, and office hours.

Beyond the conventional challenges in conducting adolescent health research, those who use emerging technology face additional issues. When studies recruit, enroll, and engage participants through electronic means, there is an inability to confirm inclusion and exclusion criteria, verify self-report measures, and compare the characteristics of those who choose to participate and/or continue through a protocol to those who are lost in the screening process and follow-up.[55]

To advance the quality of adolescent health research involving emerging technologies, I recommend that planning and implementation subscribe to the highest levels of rigor. Researchers ought to consider not only the study-plan elements, including the research question, design, subjects, measurements, analysis plan, and conclusions, but also how the introduction of technology enhances or challenges these elements. Although the delivery of protocols and messages may be novel, the foundation and configuration of research should use long-established and incorporate well-thought-out and tested methods to secure the conduct of solid work and useful findings.

REFERENCES

1. Roberts DF, Foehr UG, Rideout V. *Generation M: Media in the Lives of 8–18 Year-Olds.* Menlo Park, CA: Kaiser Family Foundation; 2005. Available at: www.kff.org/entmedia/7251.cfm. Accessed June 1, 2007
2. Lenhart A, Madden M, Hitlin P. Pew Internet & American Life Project: teens and technology— youth are leading the transition to a fully wired and mobile nation. Available at: www.pewinternet.org/pdfs/PIP_Teens_Tech_July2005web.pdf. Accessed July 27, 2005
3. Bridge Ratings. Youth spending more time with cell phones and MP3 players. Available at: www.bridgeratings.com. Accessed March 19, 2007
4. Martha C, Griffet J. Brief report: how do adolescents perceive the risks related to cell-phone use? *J Adolesc.* 2007;30:513–521
5. Lajunen HR, Keski-Rahkonen A, Pulkkinen L, Rose RJ, Rissanen A, Kaprio J. Are computer and cell phone use associated with body mass index and overweight? A population study among twin adolescents. *BMC Public Health,* 2007;7:24
6. Jung JY, Kim YC, Lin WY, Cheong PH. The influence of social environment on Internet connectedness of adolescents in Seoul, Singapore and Taipai. *New Media and Soc.* 2005;7: 64–88
7. Borzekowski DLG, Fobil JN, Asante KO. Online access by adolescents in Accra: Ghanaian teens' use of the Internet for health information. *Dev Psychol.* 2006;42:450–458
8. Ybarra ML, Kiwanuka J, Emenyonu N, Bangsberg DR. Internet use among Ugandan adolescents: implications for HIV intervention. *PLoS Med.* 2006;3:e433. Available at: http://medicine.plosjournals.org/perlserv/?request=get-document&doi=10.1371/journal.pmed.0030433
9. Foehr UG. *Media Multitasking Among American Youth: Prevalence, Predictors and Pairings.* Menlo Park, CA: Kaiser Family Foundation; 2006. Available at: www.kff.org/entmedia/upload/7592.pdf. Accessed June 1, 2007
10. Lenhart A, Madden. Social networking Web sites and teens: an overview. Pew Internet Project Data Memo. Available at: www.pewinternet.org/pdfs/PIP_SNS_Data_Memo_Jan_2007.pdf. Accessed January 7, 2007
11. Arunachalam S. Assuring quality and relevance of Internet information in the real world. *BMJ.* 1998;317:1501–1502
12. Borzekowski DLG, Rickert VI. Adolescents, the Internet and health: issues of access and content. *J Appl Dev Psychol.* 2001;22:49–59
13. Borzekowski DLG, Rickert VI. Adolescent cybersurfing for health information: a new resource that crosses barriers. *Arch Pediatr Adolesc Med.* 2001;155:813–817
14. Rideout V. *Generation rx.com: How Young People Use the Internet for Health Information.* Washington, DC: Henry J. Kaiser Family Foundation; 2001
15. Robinson Thomas N, Borzekowski, Dina LG. Effects of the SMART classroom curriculum to reduce child and family media use. *J Commun.* 2006;56:1–26
16. Borzekowski DLG, Robinson TN. The remote, the mouse, and the no. 2 pencil: the household media environment and academic achievement among third grade students. *Arch Pediatr Adolesc Med.* 2005;159:607–613
17. Roberts DF, Foehr UG. *Kids and Media in America.* New York, NY: Cambridge University Press; 2004

18. Singer DG, Singer JL, eds. *Handbook of Children and the Media.* Thousand Oaks, CA: Sage; 2000

19. Subrahmanyam K, Kraut R, Greenfield PM, Gross EF. New forms of electronic media: the impact of interactive games and the Internet on cognition, socialization, and behavior. In: Singer DL, Singer JL, eds. *Handbook of Children and the Media.* Thousand Oaks, CA: Sage; 2001: 73–99

20. Gross EF. Adolescent Internet use: what we expect, what teens report. *Appl Dev Psychol.* 2004;25:633–649

21. Turow J. *The Internet and the Family: The View From the Family, the View From the Press.* Philadelphia, PA: University of Pennsylvania, Annenberg Public Policy Center; 1999

22. Boyer EW, Shannon M, Hibberd P. The Internet and psychoactive substance use among adolescents. *Pediatrics.* 2005;115:302–305

23. Boyer EW, Lapen PT, Macalino G, Hibberd P. Dissemination of psychoactive substance information by innovative drug users. *Cyberpsychol Behav.* 2007;10:1089

24. Wilson JL, Peebles R, Hardy KK, Litt IF. Surfing for thinness: a pilot study of pro–eating disorder Web site usage in adolescents with eating disorders. *Pediatrics.* 2006;118(6). Available at: www.pediatrics.org/cgi/content/full/118/6/e1635

25. Whitlock JL, Powers JL, Eckenrode J. The virtual cutting edge: the Internet and adolescent self-injury. *Dev Psychol.* 2006;42:407–417

26. Jacobson CM, Gould M. The epidemiology and phenomenology of non-suicidal self-injurious behavior among adolescents: a critical review of the literature. *Arch Suicide Res.* 2007;11:129–147

27. Lapinski MK. StarvingforPerfect.com: a theoretically based content analysis of pro-eating disorder Web sites. *Health Commun.* 2006;20:243–253

28. Witte K. Fear control and danger control: a test of the extended parallel process model (EPPM). *Commun Monogr.* 1992;61:113–134

29. Bleakley A, Merzel CR, VanDevanter NL, Messeri P. Computer access and Internet use among urban youths. *Am J Public Health.* 2004;94:744–746

30. Yang CK, Choe BM, Baity M, Lee JH, Cho JS. SCL-90-R and 16PF profiles of senior high school students with excessive Internet use. *Can J Psychiatry.* 2005;50:407–414

31. Mitchell KJ, Finkelhor D, Wolak J. The exposure of youth to unwanted sexual material on the Internet. *Youth Soc.* 2003;34:330–358

32. Wolak J, Mitchell K, Finkelhor D. Unwanted and wanted exposure to online pornography in a national sample of youth Internet users. *Pediatrics.* 2007;119:247–257

33. Eppright T, Allwood M, Stern B, Theiss T. Internet addiction: a new type of addiction? *Mo Med.* 1999;96:133–136

34. Young KS, Rodgers RC. The relationship between depression and Internet addiction. *Cyberpsychol Behav.* 1998;1:25–28

35. Ybarra ML, Mitchell KJ, Wolak J, Finkelhor D. Examining characteristics and associated distress related to Internet harassment: findings from the Second Youth Internet Safety Survey. *Pediatrics.* 2006;118(4). Available at: www.pediatrics.org/cgi/content/full/118/4/e1169

36. Woodruff SI, Conway TL, Edwards CC, Elliott SP, Crittenden J. Evaluation of an Internet virtual world chat room for adolescent smoking cessation. *Addict Behav.* 2006; In press

37. Runge C, Lecheler J, Horn M, Tews JT, Schaefer M. Outcomes of a Web-based patient education program for asthmatic children and adolescents. *Chest.* 2006;129:581–593

38. Williamson DA, Walden HM, White MA, et al. Two-year Internet-based randomized controlled trial for weight loss in African American girls. *Obesity.* 2006;14:1231–1243

39. Puccio JA, Belzer M, Olson J, et al. The use of cell phone reminder calls for assisting HIV-infected adolescents and young adults to adhere to highly active antiretroviral therapy: a pilot study. *AIDS Patient Care STDS.* 2006;20:438–444

40. Gribble JN, Miller HG, Rogers SM, Turner CE. Interviews mode and measurement of sexual behaviors: methodological issues. *J Sex Res.* 1999;36:16–24

41. Romer D, Hornik R, Stanton B, et al. "Talking" computers: a reliable and private method to conduct interviews on sensitive topics with children. *J Sex Res.* 1997;34:3–9

42. Trapl ES, Borawski EA, Stork PP, et al. Use of audio-enhanced personal digital assistants for school-based data collection. *J Adolesc Health*. 2005;37:296–305

43. Koo M, Skinner H. Challenges of Internet recruitment: a case study with disappointing results. *J Med Internet Res*. 2005;7:e6. Available at: www.jmir.org/2005/1/e6

44. Gordon JS, Akers L, Severson HH, Danaher BG, Boles SM. Successful participant recruitment strategies for an online smokeless tobacco cessation program. *Nicotine Tob Res*. 2006;8(suppl 1):S35–S41

45. Obermayer JL, Riley WT, Asif O, Jean-Mary J. College smoking-cessation using cell phone text messaging. *J Am Coll Health*. 2004;53:71–78

46. Bersamin M, Paschall MJ, Fearnow-Kenney M, Wyrick D. Effectiveness of a Web-based alcohol-misuse and harm-prevention course among high- and low-risk students. *J Am Coll Health*. 2007;55:247–254

47. Lou C, Zhao Q, Gao E, Shah IH. Can the Internet be used effectively to provide sex education to young people in China? *J Adolesc Health*. 2006;39:720–728

48. Gilbert LK, Temby JRE, Rogers SE. Evaluating a teen STD prevention Web site. *J Adolesc Health*. 2005;37:236–242

49. Winker MA, Flanagin A, Chi-Lum B, et al. Guidelines for medical and health information sites on the Internet: principles governing AMA Websites. *JAMA*. 2000;283:1600–1601

50. Childress CA, Asamen JK. The emerging relationship of psychology and the Internet: proposed guidelines for conducting Internet intervention research. *Ethics Behav*. 1998;8:19–35

51. Buchanan T, Smith JL. Research on the Internet: validation of a World-Wide Web mediated personality scale. *Behav Res Methods Instrum Comput*. 1999;31:565–571

52. Fortson BL, Scotti JR, Del Ben KS, Chen YC. Reliability and validity of an Internet traumatic stress survey with a college student sample. *J Trauma Stress*. 2006;19:709–720

53. Raat H, Mangunkusumo RT, Landgraf JM, Kloek G, Brug J. Feasibility, reliability, and validity of ad health status measurement by the Child Health Questionnaire Child Form (CHQ-CF): Internet administration compared with the standard paper version. *Qual Life Res*. 2007;16:675–685

54. Griffiths F, Lindenmeyer A, Powell J, Lowe P, Thorogood M. Why are health care interventions delivered over the Internet? A systematic review of the published literature. *J Med Internet Res*. 2006;8:e10. Available at: www.jmir.org/2006/2/e10

55. Bull SS, McFarlane M, King D. Barriers to STD/HIV prevention on the Internet. *Health Educ Res*. 2001;16:661–670

Adolesc Med 18 (2007) 325–341

Current Research Knowledge About Adolescent Victimization via the Internet

Janis Wolak, JD[a],*, Michele L. Ybarra, MPH PhD[b],
Kimberly Mitchell, PhD[a], David Finkelhor, PhD[a]

[a]Crimes Against Children Research Center, University of New Hampshire, 10 West Edge Drive, Durham, NH 03824, USA

[b]Internet Solutions for Kids, Inc, 1820 East Garry Avenue, No. 105, Santa Ana, CA 92705, USA

In this article we review current knowledge about Internet-mediated victimization of youth, particularly as it relates to adolescents. One section addresses Internet-initiated sex crimes and online sexual solicitations, and 3 shorter sections address Internet harassment, risky online behavior, and exposure to online pornography. Although we use the term "victimization," many of the experiences we discuss do not rise to the level of criminal incidents, and many are not disturbing to the youth who are affected. For instance, 13% of youth Internet users interviewed in 2005 had been subjected to unwanted sexual solicitations in the previous year, but many of these incidents were mild and many solicitors were other youth.[1] Nonetheless, some solicitors are online child molesters who use the Internet to seek victims.[2] Internet harassment is beginning to be acknowledged as a form of bullying that, although generally not criminal, can be emotionally distressing.[3] Most online exposures to pornography among youth are not criminal events, but their impact could be serious, at least among certain vulnerable youth.[4]

We present an overview of related research, much of which was conducted by us at the Crimes Against Children Research Center (CCRC) at the University of New Hampshire. The CCRC research includes the National Juvenile Online Victimization (N-JOV) Study,† which is the only research to date that has

---

*Corresponding author.

E-mail address: Janis.Wolak@unh.edu (J. Wolak).

†In the N-JOV Study, researchers surveyed by mail a national sample of 2574 federal, state, and local law enforcement agencies about cases that involved Internet-related sex crimes against minors in which offenders were arrested during the 12 months after July 1, 2000. Researchers then conducted >600 interviews with investigators about specific cases, including those that involved Internet-initiated sex crimes, child pornography, and solicitations of undercover investigators who posed online as minors. (Data collection on a second N-JOV Study to examine changes in the rates and dynamics of such cases began in the spring of 2007.)

examined the characteristics of Internet-related sex crimes by interviewing law enforcement investigators.[5] The N-JOV Study shed light on the prevalence and dynamics of online sex crimes in which offenders were arrested by law enforcement, as well as the characteristics of victims and offenders. CCRC research also included the first and second Youth Internet Safety Surveys (YISS-1 and YISS-2), which were telephone interviews with separate national samples of youth Internet users.[1,6] These studies examined youth experiences with unwanted online sexual solicitations, exposure to pornography and harassment, and related personal Internet use and psychosocial characteristics.

INTERNET-INITIATED SEX CRIMES

Media stories about "online predators" who use the Internet to gain access to young victims have become a staple of news reports since the late 1990s, when youth Internet use became widespread. Much of the publicity about these cases has depicted online child molesters‡ who use the Internet to lure children into sexual assaults. These online molesters stereotypically portrayed by the media lurk in Internet venues that are popular with children and adolescents. They contact victims by using deception to cover up their ages and sexual intentions, tricking victims into giving out identifying information, or using information divulged in online profiles and social-networking sites. They then entice unknowing victims into meetings or stalk and abduct them. Some news reports suggest that law enforcement is facing an epidemic of sex crimes perpetrated through a new medium by a new type of criminal. However, the reality about Internet-initiated sex crimes (those in which child molesters meet victims online) is different, more complex, and possibly less frightening than the publicity about them suggests.

Research makes it clear that the stereotype of the online child molester who uses trickery and violence to assault children is inaccurate.[2,7,8] The N-JOV Study found that most Internet-initiated sex crimes involve adult male offenders who use the Internet to meet and seduce adolescents into sexual encounters.[2] The offenders use chat rooms, instant messages, and e-mail to meet potential victims. In the great majority of cases, victims are aware that they are conversing online with adults. The offenders seldom pretend to be other teens. In the N-JOV Study, only 5% of online molesters deceived victims this way. Online molesters also rarely deceive victims about their sexual interests. Sex is usually broached online, and most victims who meet offenders face-to-face go to such meetings expecting to engage in sexual activity. The offenders use Internet communications to develop intimacy with victims, many of whom profess to be in love with

---

‡Media reports, Internet-safety information, and law enforcement agencies have been using the term Internet or online "predator" to describe offenders who use the Internet to meet victims. We prefer the term "online child molester" to emphasize that most of them are not violent, and their crimes do not constitute a new type of sexual abuse but, rather, follow familiar patterns of seduction.

or feel close to their offender. When deception does occur, it often involves promises of love and romance by offenders whose intentions are purely sexual. Many victims meet face-to-face with offenders for sex more than once. Most offenders are charged with crimes such as statutory rape that involve nonforcible sexual activity with victims who are too young to consent to sexual intercourse with adults. Violence by online child molesters is rare; 5% of N-JOV Study offenders committed violent crimes, mostly rape and attempted rape.

Are Internet-Initiated Sex Crimes a New Form of Child Sexual Abuse?

Media reports and Internet-safety messages about Internet predators often suggest that online meetings between adults and youth that develop into sex crimes constitute a new type of child sexual abuse. Although a new medium for communication is involved, nonforcible sex crimes such as statutory rape are not new or uncommon. All states have laws that deem youth below a specific age (16 years in most states) too young to consent to intercourse.[9,10] Statutory rape is nonforcible by definition. In general, offenders seduce their victims. However, the degree of willingness among youthful victims may vary considerably.[10–12] These nonforcible sex crimes constitute a substantial proportion of sex crimes against minors. Analyses of crime-report data suggest that 25% of sex crimes against minors reported to police involve statutory rape, numbering an estimated 15 700 reports across the United States in 2000.[13]

How Much Are Internet-Initiated Sex Crimes Contributing to Statutory Rape?

There were ~6594 arrests nationwide for statutory rape in 2000.[13] During about the same time period (July 1, 2000, to June 30, 2001) federal, state, and local law enforcement agencies made an estimated 500 arrests for Internet-initiated sex crimes, ~95% of which were nonforcible.[2,5] This suggests that Internet-initiated sex crimes may have accounted for ~7% of statutory rapes. This proportion of arrests has almost certainly grown since 2000 as Internet use has become more widespread and more law enforcement agencies have been trained to respond to Internet-related crimes. In the context of global risk assessment, however, these numbers indicate that Internet-initiated sex crimes account for a noticeable but small proportion of statutory rape offenses and a relatively low number of the sexual offenses committed against minors overall.

What Makes Youth Vulnerable to Online Child Molesters?

Many of the media stories and much of the Internet-safety information currently available suggest that children are vulnerable to online child molesters because they are naive and inexperienced (eg, see ref 14). Such messages, which often focus on youthful loss of innocence, imply that youth will not be able to understand sexual matters they come across online and will be easily duped or fail to recognize the sexual motives of people who intend to exploit them. These messages suggest that younger youth and those who lack experience online will be particularly vulnerable, and they ignore the possibility that youth might use the Internet to pursue their own sexual interests. Nonetheless, research indicates that high school–aged youth are more likely to be victims of Internet-initiated sex crimes than preteens[2] and more likely to be sexually solicited online.[15,16] Ninety-nine percent of victims of Internet-initiated sex crimes in the N-JOV Study were 13 to 17 years old, and none were younger than 12.[2] More than 70% were high school aged (14–17 years old). Most adolescents have a fairly sophisticated understanding of the social complexities of the Internet,[17] and many engage in complex and highly interactive Internet use, which carries higher risks.[18] This is consistent with what one might expect on the basis of normal adolescent development. Adolescents are at a stage of life at which they have an intense interest in expanding their social networks, forming close relationships, and acquiring knowledge about sex.[19–21] In addition, rebellion and risky sexual behavior are hallmarks of adolescence for some youth.[22] These normal developmental factors make adolescents vulnerable to seduction and put them at risk for responding to online sexual advances from adults.[7,8]

There are several other youth characteristics in addition to age that seem to be associated with victimization by Internet-initiated sex crimes, as found in the N-JOV Study, or with receiving aggressive sexual solicitations (ie, unwanted online sexual solicitations that evolve into offline contact or threaten to do so), as examined in the YISS-1 and YISS-2.

Girls are considerably more at risk than boys for victimization by Internet-initiated sex crimes as well as for statutory rape in general.[2,11,13] They also are significantly more likely than boys to be the targets of unwanted sexual solicitations.[1]

Although girls constitute a higher proportion of victims than boys, boys who self-identify as gay or are questioning their sexual orientation may be a population that is particularly vulnerable to online victimization.[2] Boys constitute 25% of the victims in Internet-initiated sex crimes, and virtually all their offenders are male.[2] Hostility and social stigma toward homosexuality,[23,24] as well as feelings of isolation and loneliness,[25,26] may limit the face-to-face interactions of boys who self-identify as gay and their ability to form age-appropriate, intimate relationships. Concerns about confidentiality and feelings that problems are too personal to disclose may also limit their willingness to get information about sexual matters and health from trusted adults.[27] Gay boys may also turn to the Internet to meet others who are gay and find answers to questions about their sexuality, which may make them vulnerable to online child molesters.

What youth do online is also a risk factor in Internet-mediated victimization. Youth who talk online to people they do not know in person, send personal information to such people, and talk online to them about sex are more likely to receive aggressive sexual solicitations, the solicitations most likely to evolve into Internet-initiated sex crimes.[28] Moreover, it seems that the youth who engage in these types of behaviors are not typical youth Internet users. The majority of youth refrain from these behaviors[1]: two thirds do not communicate online with people they do not know in person, and approximately three quarters have not sent personal information online to such people. Only 5% report talking online to people they do not know in person about sex.

Visiting chat rooms is another characteristic associated with Internet-mediated victimization. It is related to receiving aggressive sexual solicitations, over and above the impact of communicating with, sending personal information to and talking about sex with people not known in person.[15,28] One possible explanation for the additive impact of chat-room use is that the nature of chat rooms and the kinds of interactions that occur in them create additional risk. Explicit sexual talk, sexual innuendo, and obscene language are common in unmonitored chat rooms that are geared to adolescents[29] and may attract online child molesters. Another possible explanation is that the youth who visit chat rooms are different from and more vulnerable than other youth. There is some evidence that adolescents who visit chat rooms are more likely to have problems with their parents; suffer from sadness, loneliness, or depression; have histories of sexual abuse; and engage in risky behavior than those who do not go to chat rooms.[30,31] A higher proportion of such youth may have poor judgment about online interactions or be more likely to respond to overtures from online child molesters because they are lonely, looking for parent substitutes, or interested in sexual experimentation. Chat-room use declined substantially among youth Internet users between 2000 and 2005.[1] Whether there has been a decline in online child molesters using chat rooms to locate potential victims is an open question. Some may have moved to sites that are more popular with youth, but chat rooms may still be seen as an efficient venue for locating victims if they contain a higher concentration of youth who are susceptible to sexual advances.

Another vulnerable group is youth Internet users who report offline sexual or physical abuse in the previous year. These youth are considerably more likely to receive aggressive sexual solicitations.[15,28] There are probably several mechanisms that make abused youth more vulnerable. For some, previous sexual abuse could trigger sexualized behavior that directly invites sexual advances. It could also be related to other emotional needs or developmental distortions that attract online molesters or make youth more responsive to or less aware of the inappropriateness of their advances. In addition, some abused youth are desperate for validation, rescue, or freedom from their current circumstances. They may go online looking for help and find exploiters instead.

Have Social-Networking Sites Increased the Risk of Victimization by Online Molesters?

Starting in early 2006, there was considerable publicity about the potential dangers of social-networking sites (eg, see refs 32 and 33), which have become increasingly popular with adolescents. By the end of 2006, 55% of youth aged 12 to 17 used such sites, with older girls having higher rates of use.[34] Fears among parents, child advocates, and law enforcement seem to have arisen particularly from the amount of personal information that youth may post online at networking sites. Media stories have suggested that online molesters could use information that youth post about their plans and activities to identify, locate, and stalk victims (eg, see refs 35 and 36). Nonetheless, a close perusal of media stories suggests that online molesters have not changed their tactics with the advent of social-networking sites (eg, see refs 37–39). Online molesters do not seem to be stalking unsuspecting youth but, rather, are continuing to seek youth who are susceptible to seduction. Findings from the YISS-2 suggest that maintaining online blogs or journals, which are similar to social-networking sites because they often display considerable amounts of personal information, is not associated with greater likelihood of aggressive sexual solicitation unless youth also interact online with people they do not know in person.[40] There is also evidence that two thirds of youth with social-networking pages limit access to their sites[34] and that youth are not receiving large numbers of sexual solicitations.[41] Suggestions that social-networking sites are more dangerous for youth than other types of interactive Internet use are not substantiated by the small amount of existing research on this topic.

Child-Pornography Production and Online Requests for Sexual Pictures

A feature of sexual-offending criminality that may have been facilitated by the Internet and its associated technology is child-pornography production. One in 5 online child molesters in the N-JOV Study took sexually suggestive or explicit photographs of victims or convinced victims to take such photographs of themselves or friends.[42] In the YISS-2, 4% of youth who were solicited online said they were asked to take and transmit sexual photographs of themselves.[1,43] Many of these requests seemed to constitute production of child pornography under federal statutes. In addition, if youth complied with such requests (only 1 did—a 16-year-old boy who sent a photograph to someone he believed was a 23-year-old woman), the images could easily be circulated online, and the youth pictured would not be able to retrieve them. This is a situation that some youth might not have the foresight to understand or appreciate.

Implications

Recognizing that the victims in Internet-initiated sex crimes are not young children but, rather, adolescents who are seduced into participating in nonforcible sex crimes should guide understanding of risk factors and dynamics and has implications for prevention and treatment. Simply urging parents and guardians to control, watch, or educate their children will not be effective, because adolescents are more independent and, appropriately, less supervised than younger children. Moreover, some of the most vulnerable youth may be alienated from their parents, victims of abuse, or dealing with sensitive issues such as sexual orientation that they feel their parents will not understand. Those who design prevention approaches need to acknowledge the independence and developmental interests of adolescents. It is essential to acknowledge that normal adolescent sexual feelings, urges, and curiosity are important factors in these cases. Many online child molesters are good at communicating with adolescents and understanding their emotional needs.[8] Too often approaches to prevention shy away from realistic discussions with youth about normal sexual feelings and focus on violence, which occurs rarely. By focusing on violence, advocacy groups can spread comfortable messages about child safety and innocence; adults can avoid dealing with adolescent sexuality; prevention experts and educators do not have to face the controversies that can arise in communities when sexual behavior is discussed openly and frankly; and parents do not have to confront their own discomfort about talking to their children about sex. However, the consequence is that we are not giving youth accurate information about how to recognize and respond to sexual approaches by online molesters. We recommend educating youth frankly about the dynamics of Internet-initiated and other nonforcible sex crimes as well. We need to talk to youth directly about seduction and how some adults deliberately evoke and then exploit the compelling feelings that sexual arousal can induce both online and offline. Ideally, this information would be part of a broader education program that teaches youth to recognize and avoid sexual victimization in all environments, including their homes and neighborhoods.

INTERNET HARASSMENT

Internet harassment, defined as threats or other offensive behavior sent online or posted online for others to see, is an emerging health issue related to youth Internet use.[44–48] Six percent of youth surveyed in the YISS-1 reported being harassed online,[6] and the proportion increased to 9% in the YISS-2, 5 years later.[1] Many of these incidents were mild, but 35% of harassed youth were distressed.[3]

Based on YISS-2 data, Ybarra et al[3] reported on the dynamics of harassment and the characteristics of youth who were harassed. Two thirds of harassed youth had been bothered or harassed online, in contrast to one third who had been threatened or embarrassed by someone who posted or sent messages about them for other people to see. Thus, many Internet-harassment incidents are not direct exchanges between harassers and the harassed. Approximately one third of harassed youth reported chronic online harassment (ie, ≥3 times in the previous year). Almost half of the incidents involved harassers the youth knew in person (often other youth), and approximately half of the harassers were female. Twenty-five percent of incidents spilled over into offline life because, for example, the harasser telephoned or went to the harassed youth's home.

Youth who were harassed online were disproportionately teenagers (aged 13–17) rather than preteens (aged 10–12). They were also more likely to use the Internet in certain interactive ways (ie, sending instant messages, visiting chat rooms, and keeping online journals or blogs), have borderline or clinically significant social problems, report offline interpersonal victimization, and use the Internet to harass others.[3] Although teenagers were more likely than younger youth to be harassed online, younger youth were more likely to be distressed about harassment, as were youth who reported harassment by adults (aged ≥18) and harassment that involved offline contact.

Internet harassment is occurring to ~1 in 10 youth. Almost 1 in 4 Internet harassers are 18 years of age or older, and only half are known to the harassed youth in person before the event. Because many harassed youth report incidents in which threats or offensive messages are posted online or sent to other people, advice telling youth to log off or ignore harassers does not adequately address the challenges that many youth face in responding to harassment. Practitioners who work with adolescents should partner with parents and young people to identify strategies to minimize the impact of harassment episodes based on their specific characteristics.

Using instant messages, keeping online journals or blogs, and visiting chat rooms are also associated with being harassed online. We do not recommend suggesting that youth avoid these sorts of interactive activities. Indeed, the content and tone of communications rather than the modes of transmission likely influence whether interactions are perceived as harassing. This stance is supported by findings that youth who have problems with social skills and those who use the Internet to harass others are more likely to report being harassed. Prevention efforts may be best aimed at improving online-communication skills and also coping skills, particularly among younger youth who are more likely to feel distressed about harassment.

School-based antibullying programs typically include a school-wide as well as classroom-specific focus on raising awareness and reducing acceptance of bullying behavior. The current findings suggest that antibullying interventions should also address Internet harassment by emphasizing the importance of making reports and the role that "bystanders" can play in discouraging the behavior.

RISKY ONLINE BEHAVIORS

Although many Internet-safety advocates admonish youth to refrain from posting personal information and talking to unknown people online, few have studied whether such behaviors are actually associated with risk for Internet-mediated victimization. Using data from the YISS-2, Ybarra et al[49] examined 9 potentially risky online behaviors for their relationship with online interpersonal victimization (ie, sexual solicitation and harassment): (1) posting personal information online; (2) interacting online with people not known in person; (3) having unknown people on a buddy list; (4) using the Internet to make rude and nasty comments to others; (5) sending personal information to unknown people met online; (6) downloading images from file-sharing programs; (7) visiting X-rated sites on purpose; (8) using the Internet to embarrass or harass people youth are mad at; and (9) talking online to unknown people about sex. Although these behaviors have been deemed risky, some are also quite prevalent. Just over half (56%) posted personal information online; 43% talked online to people they did not know in person; 35% had such people on their buddy list; 28% made rude or nasty comments online; 26% sent personal information online to people they did not know in person; 15% downloaded images from file-sharing programs; 13% visited X-rated Web sites on purpose; 9% used the Internet to harass or embarrass someone they were mad at; and 5% talked online to unknown people about sex.[1] Of youth Internet users aged 10 to 17, three quarters engaged in at least 1 of the 9 behaviors in the past year, and ~28% had engaged in ≥4.[49] Despite the prevalence of these behaviors, only some were individually related to online interpersonal victimization after the total number of behaviors was taken into account. Youth who used the Internet to make rude or nasty comments to others, embarrass people they were mad at multiple times, meet people online multiple ways, and talk online to unknown people about sex, along with youth who had multiple unknown people on their buddy lists, were more likely to be solicited or harassed.[49] However, displaying a pattern of risky online behavior by engaging in a number of different types of these behaviors was more important than any specific behaviors and strongly elevated the odds for solicitation or harassment. Indeed, as the number of different types of behaviors increased, so did the likelihood of online interpersonal victimization. Youth who engaged in 4 different types of risky online behavior were 11 times more likely than those with none to report online interpersonal victimization, whereas youth who engaged in 3 of these behaviors were 5 times more likely.

Sharing personal information, either by posting or actively sending it to someone online, was not by itself associated with interpersonal victimization once a youth's pattern of Internet risky behavior was taken into account. Instead, the findings of Ybarra et al[49] suggest that harassment perpetration is more strongly associated with online interpersonal victimization. Youth who harass others online by making rude or nasty comments or frequently embarrassing others are twice as likely to report an online interpersonal victimization even after adjusting for the total number of online behaviors in which they engaged.

Many types of online behaviors considered risky by educators are, for better or worse, becoming normative. For example, over half of youth Internet users have posted personal information online. Health practitioners should take this into account when assessing youth Internet use and presenting prevention information. It may not be feasible to change the entire online culture, and the promotion of prevention messages that contradict or fail to recognize widely accepted online behavior may lack credibility to youth. A harm-reduction approach may be more effective. For example, encouraging youth to restrict viewing of social-networking sites to people they know in person is probably more effective protection against unwanted sexual solicitations or harassment than admonishing them not to post personal information on such sites.

On the other hand, there may be risks associated with posting particular kinds of information or posting in particular venues. For example, youth with sexually provocative social-networking sites may be more likely to receive sexual solicitations. These youth are acting out sexually, and they may have other characteristics that explain their actions, such as histories of sexual abuse, which is associated with sexual risk-taking.[50] In these cases, the Internet may be a mode of risk transmission rather than a creator of risk. In pre-Internet days, the same youth may have frequented malls or other environments where they could meet unknown people.

The more different types of potentially risky online behaviors youth engage in, the more likely they are to be targets of online sexual solicitations and harassment. A simple checklist of the 9 behaviors documented here could help practitioners assess risk. More broadly, prevention messages should be expanded to target youth with a pattern of online risky behaviors rather than focus on specific behaviors alone. The normality of a behavior also should be taken into account. Although more than half of youth Internet users post personal information online, only 5% talk about sex with unknown people. The uniqueness of this latter behavior should be a marker for concern and intervention in and of itself. Engaging in nonnormative behaviors online, especially behaviors with sexual intent, are likely markers for other difficulties in youths' lives.

UNWANTED AND WANTED EXPOSURE TO PORNOGRAPHY

There has been extensive worry about the possible harms to youth of being exposed to online pornography.[51–53] Fueling this concern is knowledge that many youth are exposed.[1,6,54–58] Although some of this exposure is voluntary, much of it is not. In the 2005 YISS-2, 13% of youth Internet users aged 10 to 17 visited X-rated Web sites on purpose in the past year, but even more youth (34%) were exposed to online pornography they did not want to see.[1] Overall, 42% of youth Internet users aged 10 to 17 had seen online pornography in the past year, and two thirds of those reported only unwanted exposure.[4] This degree of unwanted exposure may be a new phenomenon, because before the Internet there were few places youth frequented where they might regularly encounter unsought pornography. Although there is evidence that most youth are not particularly upset when they come across pornography on the Internet,[1,54] unwanted exposure could have more of an impact than voluntary encounters. Some youth could be psychologically and developmentally unprepared for unwanted exposure, and online images may be typically more graphic and extreme than pornography available from other sources.[1,59]

Adding to concerns, unwanted exposure to online pornography has increased, rising to 34% of youth Internet users in the YISS-2 from 25% in the YISS-1, with increases among all age groups (ages 10–17) and both boys and girls.[16] Moreover, since 2000 Internet use has expanded rapidly.[60] Eighty-seven percent of youth aged 12 to 17 used the Internet in 2005, compared with 73% in 2000. These numbers suggest that millions of youth Internet users may be exposed to unwanted online pornography annually.

What Puts Youth at Risk for Unwanted Exposure to Online Pornography?

Although teenagers (aged 13–17) have higher rates of unwanted exposure than younger youth (aged 10–12), close to 20% of younger youth surveyed in the YISS-2 reported seeing online pornography that they did not want to see over the course of a year.[4,16] Wolak et al[4] found that no other demographic characteristics beside age were related to exposure, however. Amount of Internet use was not related, and online activities were not related except that youth who used file sharing to download images were more like to report unwanted exposure. This may be because pornography can be "bundled" with nonpornography downloads that youth commonly access. In addition, there were associations between unwanted exposure and offline interpersonal victimization (eg, being bullied, assaulted by peers or siblings, a victim of theft) as well as depressive symptomatology, but these associations were not strong. Youth with these latter 2 attributes may have shared some underlying common traits such as compromised judgment or impulsiveness that may explain these associations. Overall, however, it seems that much unwanted exposure arises from normal Internet use and, except for downloading images from file-sharing programs and being a teenager, is not strongly related to specific behaviors or characteristics.

Which Youth Are Most Likely to Have Wanted Exposure to Online Pornography?

Similar to offline pornography consumption, teenage boys have the highest rates of wanted exposure to online pornography.[4,58] Data from the YISS-1 suggest that youth who intentionally seek pornography are still more likely to use traditional means (eg, magazines, movies) than the Internet.[58] In the YISS-2, more than one third of male Internet users aged 16 to 17 had visited X-rated sites on purpose in the past year. Interest in sexuality is high in this age group, and among teenage boys, rates of pornography exposure were high before the advent of the

Internet.[61] Wanted exposure was also associated with talking online with un-known people about sex, using file sharing to download images, and using the Internet at friends' homes.[4] The latter may reflect a group dynamic in viewing such material.[1,61]

Delinquent tendencies and symptoms of depression were also related to wanted exposure.[4,58] There are links between delinquency and underlying tendencies for sensation seeking.[62,63] The association between wanted exposure and symptoms of depression could have a similar explanation in that some depressed youth may seek the arousal of online pornography as a means of relieving dysphoria.[64–66] These associations should not be overstated, however. Sexual curiosity among teenage boys is normal, and many might say that visiting X-rated Web sites is consistent with normal sexual development for some youth.

However, some researchers have expressed concern that exposure to online pornography during adolescence may lead to a variety of negative consequences, including undermining accepted social values and attitudes about sexual behav-ior, earlier and promiscuous sexual activity, sexual aggression, sexual deviancy, sexual offending, and sexually compulsive behavior.[53,59,61,66–69] Although it is by no means established that exposure to online or offline pornography acts as a trigger for problem sexual or other behavior among adolescents, there is evidence that pornography may increase aggression among youth with sexually aggressive tendencies.[61] If pornography can promote deviant sexual interests or offending among youth who are prone to violence, the subgroup of youth Internet users with delinquent tendencies could include the youth who are most vulnerable to such effects, given the association between juvenile sexual offending and anti-social behavior.[70] Also, some researchers have found relationships between depression and online sexually compulsive behavior.[64–66] This suggests that the group of depressed youth Internet users could contain some who might be at risk for developing online sexual compulsions that could interfere with normal sexual development or impair their ability to meet daily obligations and develop healthy relationships with peers. Much more research is needed to determine how using pornography is related to these types of problems among youth.

Reducing Exposure to Online Pornography

Filtering, blocking, or monitoring software seems effective in lowering the risk of unwanted exposure and reducing wanted exposure among youth Internet users,[4,55] although more comprehensive forms of the software seem required; simple pop-up blockers and spam filters alone did not have a preventive effect. Attending a law enforcement presentation about Internet safety was associated with reduced odds of unwanted exposure.[4] Youth may pay more attention or give more weight to information provided by law enforcement. Also, presentations may be particularly effective for a problem such as unwanted exposure, which in most cases does not seem to be an outgrowth of hard-to-change youth charac-teristics or behaviors.

Implications

Exposure to online pornography may have reached a level at which it is norma-tive among youth Internet users, particularly teenaged boys. Methodologically sound empirical research about whether and how this may be influencing youth is in order. There is some evidence that youth reactions to sexual material are diverse and complex, especially among older youth,[51] and many teens may respond thoughtfully and critically to the images they see. However, there has been very little research about the impact on youth of viewing pornography, either wanted or (more relevant) unwanted. There is no research that sheds light on whether, how, or under what circumstances unwanted exposure to pornogra-phy may trigger adverse responses in youth. Researchers in the field of sexual development do not know whether there are important "primacy effects" relating to early exposure of youth to pornography or what the effects of such exposures might be on anxieties, normative standards, or patterns of arousal in some youth. Clearly, the extent of exposure to online pornography is great enough that even if adverse effects occur to only a small fraction of youth, the numbers in absolute terms could be fairly large.

CONCLUSIONS

Responses to concerns about youth safety online can be effective only if they are based on accurate perceptions of what the safety issues are and what youth populations are impacted. New technology and periods of rapid social change often breed considerable anxiety. Sensationalized media stories and anxiety-driven stereotypes of online predators do not accurately convey the characteris-tics and dynamics of Internet-initiated sex crimes. In the rapidly changing environment created by new communications technologies, it is important that we have accurate and dispassionate information about youth behaviors, experi-ences, and their impact on health and development. Continuing research and evidence-based prevention programs are necessary to understand and effectively respond to these problems.

ACKNOWLEDGMENTS

The first Youth Internet Safety Survey was funded by the US Congress through National Center for Missing & Exploited Children grant 98MC-CX-K002. The National Juvenile Online Victimization Study and the second Youth Internet Safety Survey were funded by the National Center for Missing & Exploited Children and the Office of Juvenile Justice and Delinquency Prevention, US Department of Justice (grants 2000-JW-VX-0005, 2002-JW-BX-0002, and 2003-JN-FX-0064).

Points of view or opinions in this article are those of the authors and do not necessarily represent the official position or policies of the US Department of Justice.

REFERENCES

1. Wolak J, Mitchell K, Finkelhor D. *Online Victimization: 5 Years Later.* Alexandria, VA: National Center for Missing & Exploited Children; 2006. Available at: www.unh.edu/ccrc/pdf/CV138.pdf. Accessed July 3, 2007

2. Wolak J, Finkelhor D, Mitchell KJ. Internet-initiated sex crimes against minors: implications for prevention based on findings from a national study. *J Adolesc Health.* 2004;35:424.e11–424.e20

3. Ybarra M, Mitchell KJ, Wolak J, Finkelhor D. Risk and impact of Internet harassment: findings from the Second Youth Internet Safety Survey. *Pediatrics.* 2006;118(4). Available at: www.pediatrics.org/cgi/content/full/118/4/e1169

4. Wolak J, Mitchell KJ, Finkelhor D. Unwanted and wanted exposure to online pornography in a national sample of youth Internet users. *Pediatrics.* 2007;119:247–257

5. Wolak J, Mitchell KJ, Finkelhor D. *Internet Sex Crimes Against Minors: The Response of Law Enforcement.* Alexandria, VA: National Center for Missing & Exploited Children; 2003. Available at: www.unh.edu/ccrc/pdf/jvq/CV70.pdf. Accessed July 3, 2007

6. Finkelhor D, Mitchell KJ, Wolak J. *Online Victimization: A Report on the Nation's Youth.* Alexandria, VA: National Center for Missing & Exploited Children; 2000. Available at: www.unh.edu/ccrc/pdf/jvq/CV38.pdf. Accessed July 3, 2007

7. Berliner L. Confronting an uncomfortable reality. *APSAC Advis.* 2002;14:2–4

8. Lanning KV. Law enforcement perspective on the compliant child victim. *APSAC Advis.* 2002;14:4–9

9. Glosser A, Gardiner K, Fishman M. Statutory rape: a guide to state laws and reporting requirements: Available at: http://opa.osophs.dhhs.gov/titlex/statutory%20rape_state%20laws_lewin.pdf. Accessed July 3, 2007

10. Manlove J, Moore KA, Liechty J, Ikramullah E, Cottingham S. Sex between young teens and older individuals: a demographic portrait. Available at: www.childtrends.org/Files/StatRapeRB.pdf. Accessed July 3, 2007

11. Cheit RE, Braslow L. Statutory rape: an empirical examination of claims of "overreaction." In: Dowd N, Singer DG, Wilson RF, eds. *Handbook of Children, Culture, and Violence.* Thousand Oaks, CA: Sage; 2005

12. Darroch JE, Landry DJ, Oslak S. Age differences between sexual partners in the united states. *Fam Plann Perspect.* 1999;31:160–167

13. Troup-Leasure K, Snyder HN. Statutory rape known to law enforcement. Available at: www.ncjrs.gov/pdffiles1/ojjdp/208803.pdf. Accessed July 3, 2007

14. Kelly K. To protect the innocent, learning to keep sexual predators at bay. *U.S. News & World Report.* June 13, 2005:72–73

15. Mitchell KJ, Finkelhor D, Wolak J. Risk factors for and impact of online sexual solicitation of youth. *JAMA.* 2001;285:3011–3014

16. Mitchell KJ, Wolak J, Finkelhor D. Trends in youth reports of sexual solicitations, harassment and unwanted exposure to pornography on the Internet. *J Adolesc Health.* 2007;40:116–126

17. Yan Z. What influences children's and adolescents' understanding of the complexity of the Internet? *Dev Psychol.* 2006;42:418–428

18. Livingstone S. Drawing conclusions from new media research: reflections and puzzles regarding children's experience of the Internet. *Inform Soc.* 2006;22:219–230

19. Buhrmester D. Need fulfilment, interpersonal competence, and the developmental contexts of early adolescent friendship. In: Bukowski WM, Newcomb AF, Hartup WW, eds. *The Company They Keep: Friendship in Childhood and Adolescence.* Cambridge, United Kingdom: Cambridge University Press; 1996:158–185

20. Collins WA, Laursen B. Conflict and relationships during adolescence. In: Uhlinger Shantz C, Hartup WW, eds. *Conflict in Child and Adolescent Development.* Cambridge, United Kingdom: Cambridge University Press; 1992:216–241

21. DeLamater J, Friedrich WN. Human sexual development. *J Sex Res.* 2002;39:10–14

22. Jessor R. New perspectives on adolescent risk behavior. In: Jessor R, ed. *New Perspectives on Adolescent Risk Behavior.* New York, NY: Cambridge University Press; 1998:1–10

23. Tharinger D, Wells G. An attachment perspective on the developmental challenges of gay and lesbian adolescents: the need for continuity of caregiving from family and schools. *School Psychol Rev.* 2000;29:158–172

24. Williams T, Connolly J, Pepler D, Craig W. Peer victimization, social support, and psychosocial adjustment of sexual minority adolescents. *J Youth Adolesc.* 2005;34:471–482

25. Martin JI, D'Augelli AR. How lonely are gay and lesbian youth? *Psychol Rep.* 2003;93:486

26. Sullivan M. Social alienation in gay youth. *J Hum Behav Soc Environ.* 2002;5:1–17

27. Dubow EF, Lovko KR, Kausch DF. Demographic differences in adolescents' health concerns and perceptions of helping agents. *J Clin Child Psychol.* 1990;19:44–54

28. Mitchell KJ, Finkelhor D, Wolak J. Youth Internet users at risk for the most serious online sexual solicitations. *Am J Prev Med.* 2007;32:532–537

29. Subrahmanyam K, Smahel D, Greenfield P. Connecting developmental constructions to the Internet: identity presentation and sexual exploration in online teen chat rooms. *Dev Psychol.* 2006;42:395–406

30. Beebe TJ, Asche SE, Harrison PA, Quinlan KB. Heightened vulnerability and increased risk-taking among adolescent chat room users: results from a statewide school survey. *J Adolesc Health.* 2004;35:116–123

31. Sun P, Unger JB, Palmer PH, et al. Internet accessibility and usage among urban adolescents in southern California: implications for Web-based health research. *Cyberpsychol Behav.* 2005;8: 441–453

32. Apuzzo M. Prosecutors: men used MySpace.com to meet underage girls for sex. *The Boston Globe.* March 2, 2006. Available at: www.boston.com/news/local/connecticut/articles/2006/03/02/prosecutors_men_used_myspacecom_to_meet_underage_girls_for_sex. Acessed July 3, 2007

33. Bahney A. Don't talk to invisible strangers. *The New York Times.* March 9, 2006:G1

34. Lenhart A, Madden. Social networking Web sites and teens: an overview. Pew Internet Project Data Memo. Available at: www.pewinternet.org/pdfs/PIP_SNS_Data_Memo_Jan_2007.pdf. Accessed July 3, 2007

35. Kornblum J. Social Websites scrutinized; MySpace, others reviewed in crimes against teenagers. *USA Today.* February 13, 2006;6D

36. Roeper R. Wide-open MySpace.com filled with teens, danger. *Chicago Sun Times.* April 12, 2006;Sect 11:1

37. Gustafson P. Offender admits sex with girl, 15. *Minneapolis Star Tribune.* February 16, 2006;5B

38. Rawe J. How safe is MySpace? *Time.* July 3, 2006:34–36

39. Schrobsdorff S. Q&A: how to keep teens safe on MySpace.com. *Newsweek.* January 27, 2006. Available at: www.msnbc.msn.com/id/11065951/site/newsweek. Accessed July 3, 2007

40. Mitchell KJ, Wolak J, Finkelhor D. Are blogs putting youth at risk for online sexual solicitation or harassment? *Child Abuse Negl.* 2007; In press

41. Rosen L. Adolescents in MySpace: identity formation, friendship and sexual predators. Available at: www.csudh.edu/psych/Adolescents%20in%20MySpace%20-%20Executive%20Summary.pdf. Accessed July 3, 2007

42. Wolak J, Finkelhor D, Mitchell KJ. The varieties of child pornography production. In: Taylor M, Quayle E, eds. *Viewing Child Pornography on the Internet.* Dorset, United Kingdom: Russell House Publishing; 2005:31–48

43. Mitchell KJ, Finkelhor D, Wolak J. Online requests for sexual pictures of youth: risk factors and incident characteristics. *J Adolesc Health.* 2007; In press

44. Berson IR, Berson MJ, Ferron JM. Emerging risks of violence in the digital age: lessons for educators from an online study of adolescent girls in the United States. *J Sch Violence.* 2002;1:51–71

45. Hinduja S, Patchin JW. Offline consequences of online victimization: school violence and delinquency. *J Sch Violence.* 2007; In press

46. Keith S, Martin ME. Cyber-bullying: creating a culture of respect in a cyber world. *Reclaiming Child Youth.* 2005;13:224–228

47. Patchin JW, Hinduja S. Bullies move beyond the schoolyard: a preliminary look at cyberbullying. *Youth Violence Juv Justice.* 2006;4:148–169

48. Tettegah SY, Betout D, Taylor KR. Cyber-bullying and schools in an electronic era. In: Tettegah S, Hunter R, eds. *Issues in Administration, Policy and Applications in K12 School.* Vol 8. London, United Kingdom: Elsevier; 2006:17–28

49. Ybarra ML, Mitchell KJ, Wolak J, Finkelhor D. Internet prevention messages: targeting the right online behaviors? *Arch Pediatr Adolesc Med.* 2007;161:138–145

50. Raj A, Silverman JG, Amaro H. The relationship between sexual abuse and sexual risk among high school students: findings from the 1997 Massachusetts Youth Risk Behavior Survey. *Matern Child Health J.* 2000;4:125–134

51. Cantor J, Mares ML, Hyde JS. Autobiographical memories of exposure to sexual media content. *Media Psychol.* 2003;5:1–31

52. Escobar-Chaves S, Tortolero S, Markham C, Low B, Eitel P, Thickstun P. Impact of the media on adolescent sexual attitudes and behaviors. *Pediatrics.* 2005;116:303–326

53. Greenfield PM. Inadvertent exposure to pornography on the Internet: implication of peer-to-peer file-sharing networks for child development and families. *Appl Dev Psychol.* 2004;25:741–750

54. Livingstone S, Bober M. *United Kingdom Children Go Online: Surveying the Experiences of Young People and Their Parents.* London, United Kingdom: London School of Economics and Political Science; 2004

55. Mitchell KJ, Finkelhor D, Wolak J. The exposure of youth to unwanted sexual material on the Internet: a national survey of risk, impact, and prevention. *Youth Soc.* 2003;34:330–358

56. Peter J, Valkenburg PM. Adolescents' exposure to sexually explicit material on the Internet. *Commun Res.* 2006;33:178–204

57. Rideout V. *Generation rx.com: How Young People Use the Internet for Health Information.* Washington, DC: Henry J. Kaiser Family Foundation; 2001

58. Ybarra ML, Mitchell KJ. Exposure to Internet pornography among children and adolescents: a national survey. *Cyberpsychol Behav.* 2005;8:473–486

59. Thornburgh D, Lin H, eds. *Youth, Pornography, and the Internet.* Washington, DC: National Academy Press; 2002

60. Lenhart A, Madden M, Hitlin P. Pew Internet & American Life Project: teens and technology—youth are leading the transition to a fully wired and mobile nation. Available at: www.pewinternet.org/pdfs/PIP_Teens_Tech_July2005web.pdf. Accessed July 3, 2007

61. Malamuth N, Huppin M. Pornography and teenagers: the importance of individual differences. *Adolesc Med Clin.* 2005;16:315–326

62. Martin C, Kelly T, Rayens M, et al. Sensation seeking and symptoms of disruptive disorder: association with nicotine, alcohol, and marijuana use in early and mid-adolescence. *Psychol Rep.* 2004;94:1075–1082

63. Moore S, Rosenthal D. Venturesomeness, impulsiveness, and risky behavior among older adolescents. *Percept Mot Skills.* 1993;76:98

64. Black DW, Belsare G, Schlosser S. Clinical features, psychiatric comorbidity, and health-related quality of life in persons reporting compulsive computer use behavior. *J Clin Psychiatry.* 1999;60:839–844

65. Cooper A, Delmonico DL, Griffin-Shelley E, Mathy RM. Online sexual activity: an examination of potentially problematic behaviors. *Sex Addict Compulsivity.* 2004;11:129–143

66. Cooper A, Putnam DE, Planchon LA, Boies SC. Online sexual compulsivity: getting tangled in the net. *Sex Addict Compulsivity.* 1999;6:79–104

67. Kanuga M, Rosenfeld WD. Adolescent sexuality and the Internet: the good, the bad, and the URL. *J Pediatr Adolesc Gynecol.* 2004;17:117–124

68. Rich M. Sex screen: the dilemma of media exposure and sexual behavior. *Pediatrics.* 2005;116: 329–331

69. Zillmann D. Influence of unrestrained access to erotica on adolescents' and young adults' dispositions toward sexuality. *J Adolesc Health.* 2000;27:41–44

70. Righthand S, Welch C. *Juveniles Who Have Sexually Offended: A Review of the Professional Literature*. Washington, DC: Office of Juvenile Justice and Delinquency Prevention; 2001. Available at: www.ncjrs.gov/pdffiles1/ojjdp/184739.pdf. Accessed July 3, 2007

Adolesc Med 18 (2007) 342–356

Application of Interactive, Computer Technology to Adolescent Substance Abuse Prevention and Treatment

Lisa A. Marsch, PhD[a,b,*], Warren K. Bickel, PhD[b,c], Michael J. Grabinski, MCSD[b,d]

[a]*Center for Drug Use and HIV Research, National Development and Research Institutes, 71 West 23rd Street, 8th Floor, New York, NY 10010, USA*

[b]*HealthSim, LLC, 101 West 23rd Street, Room 525, New York, NY 10011, USA*

[c]*Center for Addiction Research, University of Arkansas for Medical Sciences, 4301 West Markham Street, Little Rock, AR 72205, USA*

[d]*Red 5 Group, LLC, 10 Hanover Square, Room 11G, New York, NY 10005, USA*

Substance use among youth remains a major public health problem. Almost half (48%) of all 12th-graders have tried an illicit drug in their lifetime. More than 42% of this same age group have tried marijuana, 8% have tried cocaine, 1.4% report heroin use, and 4.4% report methamphetamine use in their lifetime. More than 72% of this same age group have used alcohol, and >56% have been drunk. In addition, >47% of this group have used cigarettes.[1] Moreover, rates of abuse of prescription painkillers (opioids) among adolescents have been estimated to have increased ~542% in the past decade.[2] A recent survey conducted by the Partnership for a Drug-Free America[3] with youth in grades 7 to 12 reported that ~1 (18%) in 5 teenagers reported having abused Vicodin (hydrocodone/acetaminophen), and 1 (10%) in 10 teenagers reported having abused OxyContin (a controlled-release form of oxycodone hydrochloride).

Substance use at an early age may increase the likelihood of using other drugs,[4] increase risky behavior (eg, alcohol-related accidents, risky sexual behavior), and lead to poor educational outcomes that may have long-lasting negative personal and economic consequences such as school dropout, delinquency, and difficulty in making the transition to adulthood.[5,6] In addition, risk behavior that is often associated with substance use among adolescents increases the risk of unintended pregnancies and contracting and spreading sexually transmitted infections (STIs), hepatitis, HIV, and other serious diseases.[7,8]

---

*Corresponding author.
E-mail address: marsch@ndri.org (L. A. Marsch).

Fortunately, a number of effective substance abuse–prevention and –treatment interventions for youth exist. Many prevention and treatment programs generally focus on developing the skills necessary to resist peer, family, and other social influences that promote drug use. Treatment programs for youth often also focus on promoting skills training to eliminate situations that are precursors to drug use and increase activities that are incompatible with or unrelated to drug use. In addition, effective prevention and treatment programs generally provide more generalized skills training that is necessary for social competency and the ability to cope with stressful life situations. These programs are designed to enhance decision-making, problem-solving, communication, and self-management skills.[9-12]

Although such effective prevention and treatment programs for youth exist, delivery of these interventions is often challenging. Such challenges include limited financing for providing prevention and treatment, slow adoption of science-based innovations, and difficulty in ensuring the fidelity of science-based interventions. In addition, many existing interventions generally do not use interactive, activity-oriented, methodologies for effective knowledge promotion and skills training. Moreover, the availability of services may not fully meet demand in some areas, including rural communities in which access to care may be limited.[13-16]

These challenges to current prevention and treatment efforts support the need to disseminate science-based, efficacious drug abuse interventions that are cost-effective, require limited educator or therapist training, and allow the intervention to be applied with fidelity.

Our group has been involved in a number of research-and-development activities that are focused on the application of informational technologies to adolescent substance abuse prevention and treatment. Applying informational technologies to the delivery of science-based interventions may allow for unique opportunities to provide widespread dissemination of cost-effective interventions with consistency and in a manner that is engaging and acceptable to youth. Indeed, most adolescents regularly use computers in a variety of settings; thus, the computer would likely be a highly acceptable medium for interventions with youth. Eighty-seven percent of 12- to 17-year-olds go online at home at least once monthly.[17] Youth also have access to a wide range of technology tools at school that would enable them to effectively use computer-based programs. More than 92% of US public schools have Internet access, and >75% have high-speed Internet access. Seventy-eight percent of schools in 1 study reported that the majority of their teachers use computers daily, often for instructional purposes.[18] Thus, computerized substance abuse–related interventions could be implemented in most US public schools. Moreover, in addition to their use in the home and at school, computer-based interventions for youth could be used in a variety of settings including after-school programs, community-based organizations, and health care provider offices.

Many students report that they find interactive computer learning environments to be preferable to traditional learning environments in that computer-based learning provides the opportunity for active and independent problem solving and individualized instruction.[19,20] Also, computer-based learning may appeal to students who normally resist other forms of learning.[21,22]

CASE STUDY: COMPUTER-BASED PREVENTION AND TREATMENT PROGRAMS FOR YOUTH

Here we provide an overview of 2 interactive, computer-based substance abuse–prevention and –treatment interventions that we have developed for adolescents to date. These programs include:

1. *HeadOn: Substance Abuse Prevention for Grades 6–8*, an interactive, substance abuse–prevention multimedia program for middle school–aged youth; and
2. a customizable, interactive program focused on prevention of HIV, hepatitis, and STIs among youth in substance abuse treatment.

We ensured that the content in each of these programs is evidence based and grounded in a scientific understanding of the types of skills and information that are critical for effective prevention. In addition, we designed these programs to use several evidence-based informational technologies that have been shown to be critical in effectively training key skills and information. All of these programs are browser based and can be delivered via the Internet or packaged in a CD-ROM. We designed these programs to have such flexibility in their deployment so that they can be used in a variety of settings.

Core Informational Technologies

We use a variety of multimedia elements in our prevention and treatment programs for youth. As described in more detail in the next section, these elements include a variety of interactive exercises to better enhance learning and personalize content for program users, interactive worksheets with response-specific feedback and suggestions, interactive games, and graphics and animation to better illustrate certain concepts or skills. In addition, all of our programs include 2 key computer-based technologies: fluency-based, computer-assisted instruction (CAI) and computer simulation technologies to train relevant skills and information.

Fluency-Based CAI

We created a CAI engine that incorporates fluency-building methodologies, and we have included it in each of our substance abuse–prevention and –treatment programs for youth. CAI programs, which use the computer as a medium of instruction, can selectively present information, require active responding by a computer user to queries that are designed to assess knowledge acquisition, and evaluate and provide immediate feedback to the user's responses.[23,24] Fluency-based CAI is an educational technology that is based on the precision teaching/overlearning literature[25] and requires the learner to develop a predetermined level of accuracy and speed in responding during an active learning process.

In this process, a computer user is presented with the information to be learned on the computer screen, and the user controls the rate of presentation of information. After all information has been presented, the user is presented with a series of multiple-choice questions followed by a series of fill-in-the-blank questions that they are required to answer. Multiple permutations of each question are presented to train a given concept to mastery. As a user develops greater knowledge about a given topic and becomes increasingly fluent in the information provided on that topic, he or she should be able to read and respond accurately to the questions at increasingly faster rates. Thus, read and response times for each question change continuously as training progresses. If a user responds correctly to a question, both the read and response times for that question decrease on the next presentation of that question. Conversely, if a user responds incorrectly to a question, both the read and response times for that question increase on the next presentation of that question. Users are given immediate feedback on all responses. A question is no longer presented after a predetermined "mastery" criterion is reached (eg, correct responses made on 3 consecutive presentations of a question and the final criterion response time for the question is attained). As a result, the content of the CAI program is adjusted on the basis of an individual user's level of responding.

By training individuals to reach preestablished behavioral fluency criteria, CAI programs have been demonstrated to promote "mastery" of a specific behavior along with short-term and long-term retention of knowledge on a given topic.[26,27] The use of performance feedback, hints, and remediation in computer-based learning functions as a "computer-based coach" by allowing users to evaluate their own progress and, in so doing, become better equipped to learn from their errors.[28] We have used CAI technology in our computer-based prevention and treatment interventions to effectively promote long-term retention of key skills and information that are important in effective interventions in these groups.[13,29,30]

Computer-Based Simulation

We also use various types of simulation technologies in our prevention and treatment programs for youth. Simulations place the user in a realistic task environment where he or she may continually interact with, and receive feedback from, an active and complex social or physical system that mimics, or is only marginally abstracted from, the real world. Furthermore, time and space may be compressed within simulated environments, which enables the user to experiment with alternative behavioral choices and thereby contact both the short-term and long-term outcomes associated with such choices without having to make such choices within a real-world setting.[31] In some of our programs, we include interactive videos that present actors modeling various behaviors for the program user to better learn the modeled behavior (eg, how to be assertive, how to make good decisions). They also create experiential learning environments that simulate real-world experiences and thereby enable the exploration of a wide variety of "what-if" scenarios while providing far more specific feedback than that provided by role-playing situations (eg, effective drug-refusal skills, effective communication skills).[23–32]

By combining the explicit instruction provided by the CAI and fluency-building technology with the experiential learning provided by simulation technology, a learner may exhibit "true mastery" of material and establish a "permanent repertoire" of behavior based on the learning process.[23,33] CAI and computer simulation technologies, when presented within the context of a multimedia computer-based learning program, enable multimodality (integration of text, pictures, video, etc) and interactivity.[34–36] As such, computer-based learning programs can be easily exported and applied with fidelity.

HeadOn: Substance Abuse Prevention for Grades 6–8

Our group developed a computer-based, substance abuse–prevention program, *HeadOn: Substance Abuse Prevention for Grades 6–8* (available at www.preventionsciencemedia.com).[30] This program is based on the components of primary prevention efforts that have shown to be efficacious in preventing initiation to drug use and are presented by using technologies that have been shown to be effective in teaching and promoting long-term retention of skills and information. Focus groups of middle school–aged youth provided input and feedback at all stages of development of this program.

HeadOn is composed of several simulated neighborhoods in which youth can go to learn important information about drug abuse prevention. An animated cab driver-narrator takes the youth to the neighborhoods of their choice, and they can choose to interact with various locations in the neighborhood (eg, house, school, ambulance driving on a neighborhood street) to learn about issues important to science-based drug abuse prevention. These topics include (1) the various classes of drugs and their immediate and long-term physiologic and behavioral effects; (2) the risks of experimentation with drugs; (3) the potential consequences of drug use; (4) a cost/benefit reasoning strategy that youth can use to effectively respond to drug offers; (5) drug-refusal skills training; (6) risk of misusing prescription drugs; (7) how to effectively understand and resist advertisements for licit drugs; (8) misconceptions many youth have in which they tend to overestimate the percentage of their peers who use drugs; (9) social-skills training (eg, effective communication skills); and (10) self-management skills training. Each location where a given topic is addressed includes an interactive video in which youth can make decisions for characters acting out a scenario that is relevant to the topic addressed at that location, and they can explore the various consequences of decisions they make. Also, each location includes a CAI section that trains youth to fluency levels of key information important to drug abuse prevention. As youth complete the CAI sections of *HeadOn*, they earn skills cards, which they can use in an electronic card game called *Skills Challenge*. In the game, youth can play against various challengers who present them with a series of challenges that fall under 5 main categories that are thematically related to the categories of skills youth learned about in the program (decision-making, drug refusal, media, social and self-management skills). Youth must select the appropriate skills cards from their deck of cards to best respond to challengers. All program sections are graphically rich and highly interactive. Sample screen shots from this program are included in Figs 1 and 2.

We evaluated the relative efficacy of the *HeadOn* program compared with the Life Skills Training drug abuse–prevention curriculum, a curriculum of demonstrated effectiveness,[37,38] in a school-based evaluation across 4 middle schools ($N = 272$). Students in 2 of the schools received substance abuse–prevention training via the *HeadOn* computer-based prevention program over the course of 15 sessions during the school year. Students in the 2 other schools received

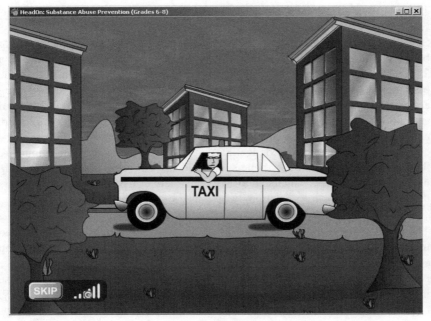

Fig 1. Introduction to cab driver-narrator in *HeadOn: Substance Abuse Prevention 6–8*.

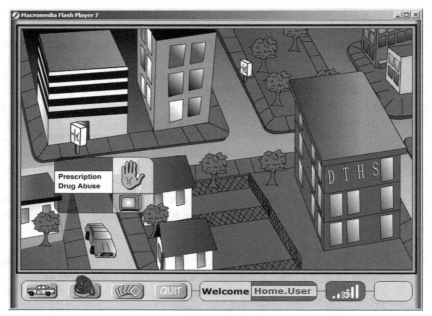

Fig 2. Example of a neighborhood within *HeadOn: Substance Abuse Prevention for Grades 6–8.*

substance abuse–prevention training via the demonstrably efficacious Life Skills Training program over the course of 15 sessions.

Student participants in all schools completed a battery of questionnaires both before and after their prevention training. Specifically, participants completed a 25-item, multiple-choice knowledge assessment, which objectively measured the participants' level of accurate knowledge on content important to effective drug abuse–prevention programs. Knowledge was assessed regarding the effects of substance use, perceived prevalence of use among the participants' peer group, and advertising knowledge, as well as decision-making, drug-refusal, communication, and social-skills knowledge. Participants also completed a questionnaire that assessed their attitudes, beliefs, intentions, and behavior related to drug use.[39] This measure was included to assess a variety of risk and protective factors that have been shown to be strongly associated with substance use.[40,41]

The results demonstrate that, although students in both groups showed marked increases in knowledge about drug abuse prevention after their intervention compared with baseline, those in the *HeadOn* group had a significantly higher percent accuracy (77%) on this measure after their training compared with those in the Life Skills group (64%) (test of differential change in percent accuracy: $t_{249} = 6.52$; $P = .0001$). Also, participants in the *HeadOn* and Life Skills groups generally achieved comparable, positive outcomes after completing their prevention intervention on a wide variety of measures, including actual self-reported rates of both cigarettes and alcohol use, intentions to use substances, attitudes toward substances, beliefs about prevalence of substance use among both their peers and adults, and likelihood of refusing a drug offer.

Importantly, *HeadOn* was well liked by the youth. Youth who evaluated the program reported that the computer program was highly useful (mean: 73.23 of 100 points). Also, participants reported that they learned a great deal about what to do when offered a drug from the computer program (mean: 75.03 of 100). They also reported that the computer-based program was highly interesting (mean: 76.01 of 100) and fun (mean: 73.58 of 100). In addition, teachers who used the computer program reported that they thought the computer program was highly useful in providing drug abuse prevention in the classroom. For example, 1 teacher said, "I liked the fact that I could help out individual students while others were working. I liked being able to have students move along at their own rate." One teacher who used Life Skills said, "I don't feel that Life Skills should be the only drug prevention program used in schools. I was frustrated that the Life Skills trainers told us that the curriculum must be implemented exactly the way they required because this is not always practical to do given other demands on our time in the classroom." Importantly, a cost analysis demonstrated that the *HeadOn* program produced slightly greater accuracy in drug abuse prevention–related knowledge at a little more than half the cost of the Life Skills Training program.

These findings demonstrate that effective prevention science can be delivered successfully via a multimedia system. Use of this efficacious, computerized substance abuse–prevention program by middle school–aged youth may markedly expand the reach of science-based substance abuse prevention. *HeadOn* has been deemed a "promising program" by a panel of independent reviewers and is included in a repository of science-based prevention programs in the National Registry of Effective Programs and Practices sponsored by the Substance Abuse and Mental Health Services Administration.

Computer-Based Prevention of HIV, Hepatitis, and STIs Among Youth

We developed and examined the feasibility and efficacy of an interactive, computer-assisted HIV-, STI-, and disease-prevention program for youth in substance abuse treatment that incorporates effective components of both prevention science and educational technologies.

The program was designed for youth in substance abuse treatment, because youth who use drugs are at particularly high risk for infection with HIV, STIs, and other similarly contracted infections. Compared with their non–drug-using peers, adolescents who use drugs report engaging in significantly more behaviors that place them at risk for infection with these diseases.[42] Specifically, drug-using adolescents report having sexual intercourse at an earlier age, having higher numbers of sexual partners, using condoms less frequently, and engaging in different types of risk behavior (eg, prostitution for drugs, money, or shelter) compared with their non–drug-using peers. In addition, youth who use drugs are shown to have less HIV-related knowledge, lower perceived susceptibility to HIV infection, higher levels of impulsivity, and less self-efficacy to engage in preventive behavior.[43,44]

The majority of substance-abusing youth who become infected with HIV and other serious diseases contract them through risky sexual behavior that may be indirectly related to their drug-use behavior.[45] Indeed, substance use impairs decision-making and is linked with risk for HIV infection more often for youth than for adults.[46,47] In addition, some drugs, such as injected cocaine, smoked cocaine (crack), and amphetamines, may heighten perceptions of sexual arousal and promote high-risk sexual activity.[48,49] Substance-abusing youth may also become infected with HIV or other diseases with similar transmission dynamics through injection-drug use. This group may be at risk from both risky drug-injection practices (eg, needle sharing), as well as high-risk sexual behavior (eg, often to obtain drugs or to obtain money used to secure drugs).[50–52]

Although several age-appropriate and effective interventions have been identified for young substance abusers, most interventions have been narrow in focus and are generally not structured to readily address changing patterns of drug use among adolescents that place them at risk for infection with HIV, STIs, and similarly transmitted diseases.[45] In addition, most adolescent substance abuse–treatment programs do not routinely offer effective HIV-, STI-, or hepatitis-prevention interventions. Thus, this computer-delivered prevention program was designed to fill this gap in services by offering a comprehensive and flexible prevention tool that may be modified for use with various subpopulations of young substance abusers with specific risk factors for infection with HIV and other serious diseases.

This self-directed program is composed of age-appropriate content that is delivered across 25 program modules that address important drug- and sex-related factors that may place young substance abusers at risk for HIV, STIs, or other serious diseases. The modules provide information about HIV, hepatitis, and STIs, teach how alcohol and other substance abuse may increase one's risk for contracting various infections/diseases, information on risk reduction (eg, selecting and correctly using condoms, identifying and managing triggers for risky sexual behavior or drug use), and teach relevant skills (eg, decision-making skills, negotiation skills). In addition, several modules were developed specifically for youth who may be infected with hepatitis or with HIV. The program also includes a customization program that is used to tailor the program to meet the unique prevention needs of a given adolescent. In this process, youth will complete a computerized assessment. The program will then suggest which modules may be relevant to a given adolescent and the order in which they may access the modules on the basis of their risk profile of responses on the assessment. This customization feature considers alcohol and other substance use, intentions to use alcohol and other substances, injection-drug use, and whether a youth may be infected with HIV and/or hepatitis. Sample screen shots from this program are provided in Figs 3 and 4.

Feedback sessions that we conducted with adolescents indicated that the program produced marked increases in accurate knowledge and skills regarding HIV, hepatitis, and STI prevention (from baseline levels of 50%–65% accuracy to 95%–100% accuracy after youth completed the program modules). Also, youth ranked the computer-based program as very easy to understand (mean: 90 of 100 points), highly useful (mean: 80 of 100 points), and highly likeable (mean: 80 of 100 points). They also rated the program as "much better" than other education they had received on this topic in adolescent treatment programs (mean: 85 of 100 points).

We conducted a controlled trial to evaluate the effectiveness of including this program as part of an enhanced prevention intervention for adolescents in substance abuse treatment compared with a standard-of-care comparison group ($n = 56$, 28 per group). Youth in the enhanced-condition group completed their customized program on the computer system and participated in a single-group educational session that was led by a prevention specialist, whereas those in the standard-condition group only participated in the educational group. On average, the youth in the enhanced intervention completed their customized program on the computer system in ~2 to 4 hours.

Youth in both study conditions completed a number of measures of HIV/disease-prevention knowledge, actual rates of substance use, intentions to use substances, and attitudes about safer sex before completing their respective prevention intervention as well as 1, 2, and 4 months after completing the intervention.

Both groups reported significant increases in their intentions to use condoms during sex and in their perception of the importance of carefully choosing sex partners and limiting their number of sex partners. In addition, both groups reported significantly more positive attitudes about engaging in safer sex (all P values were <.05). In addition, the enhanced condition promoted significantly greater increases in HIV/disease-prevention knowledge at all postinterventions relative to the standard condition (time effect: $P < .0001$; group by time: $P = .001$). The enhanced condition also promoted significantly greater increases in self-reported risk for HIV (group effect: $P < .001$) and was perceived as significantly more useful ($P = .02$) relative to the standard condition. These data suggest this computer-based program may be an effective, engaging intervention for youth and may increase the adoption of effective HIV- and disease-prevention science for a variety of adolescent subpopulations of at-risk youth.

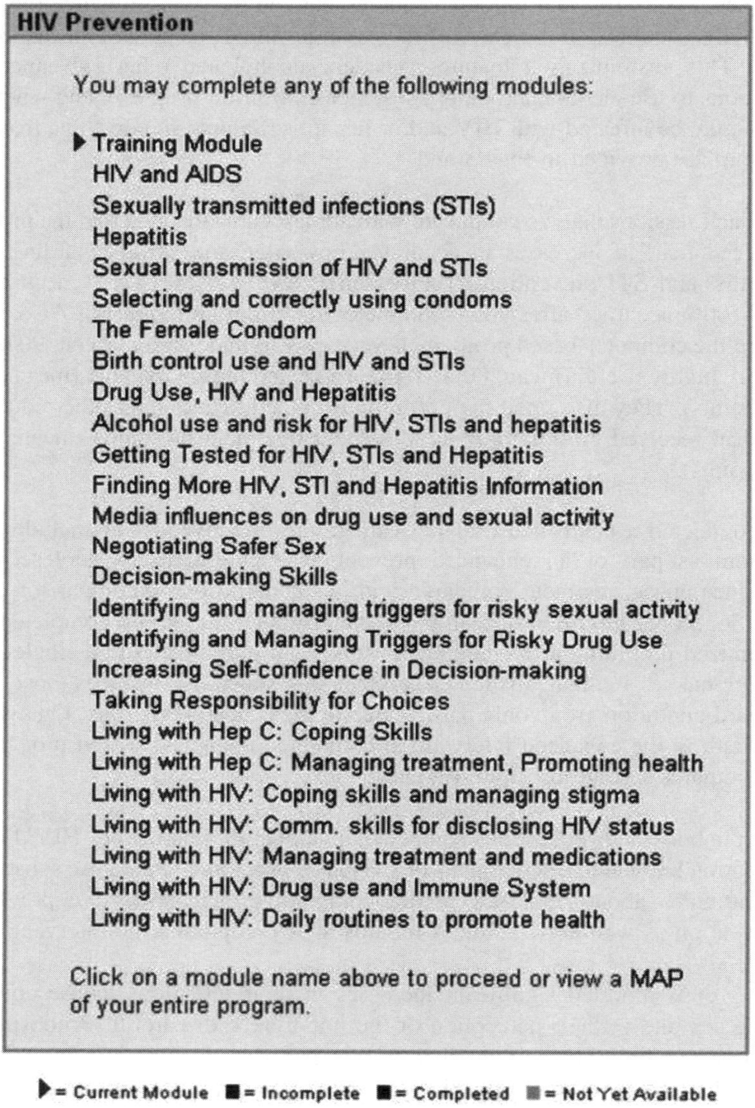

HIV Prevention

You may complete any of the following modules:

▶ Training Module
HIV and AIDS
Sexually transmitted infections (STIs)
Hepatitis
Sexual transmission of HIV and STIs
Selecting and correctly using condoms
The Female Condom
Birth control use and HIV and STIs
Drug Use, HIV and Hepatitis
Alcohol use and risk for HIV, STIs and hepatitis
Getting Tested for HIV, STIs and Hepatitis
Finding More HIV, STI and Hepatitis Information
Media influences on drug use and sexual activity
Negotiating Safer Sex
Decision-making Skills
Identifying and managing triggers for risky sexual activity
Identifying and Managing Triggers for Risky Drug Use
Increasing Self-confidence in Decision-making
Taking Responsibility for Choices
Living with Hep C: Coping Skills
Living with Hep C: Managing treatment, Promoting health
Living with HIV: Coping skills and managing stigma
Living with HIV: Comm. skills for disclosing HIV status
Living with HIV: Managing treatment and medications
Living with HIV: Drug use and Immune System
Living with HIV: Daily routines to promote health

Click on a module name above to proceed or view a MAP
of your entire program.

▶ = Current Module   ■ = Incomplete   ■ = Completed   ■ = Not Yet Available

Fig 3. Screen from the HIV-, hepatitis-, and STI-prevention program showing a list of module topics.

CONCLUSIONS

Our evaluations of computer-based substance abuse–prevention and –treatment interventions for youth to date have underscored the effectiveness of such interventions in producing desired health-behavior change. Computer-based in-

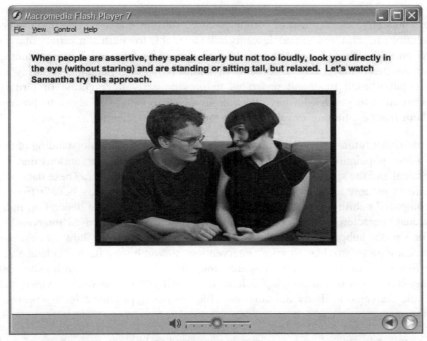

Fig 4. Sample video still from the HIV-, hepatitis-, and STI-prevention program modeling effective negotiation skills.

terventions for youth may be useful as stand-alone programs or as supplements to more-traditional interventions. Our comparisons of computer-delivered to person-delivered interventions have generally produced comparable outcomes, which may be particularly meaningful in environments where resources for intervention delivery may be limited. As demonstrated in our preliminary cost analyses, delivery of such computer-based interventions may also be cost-effective, because a computer-based program can be used numerous times with most of its expense associated with the 1-time purchase of hardware and software, whereas the cost of the person-delivered intervention is typically a fixed cost per use. We are currently conducting formal cost-effectiveness analyses to systematically examine this issue.

Importantly, as supported by our research experience, computer-based interventions are highly acceptable to youth. This may be particularly true when sensitive topics such as substance abuse and sexual behavior are addressed. Because of their self-guided, highly interactive nature and the anonymity they afford, computer-based interventions may provide engaging and effective tools for youth. In addition, they may be particularly useful in that they can be readily modified to accommodate new information as it becomes available.

In our ongoing research and development of computer-based interventions, we are pursuing development of computer-based substance abuse–prevention interventions for children and adolescents to be available to youth at a variety of ages to ensure access to science-based, age-appropriate prevention programming across the course of development. In addition, we are planning an array of computer-based treatment programs to provide early intervention or tertiary prevention to youth who have become involved in substance abuse to prevent them from continuing to follow a substance-abusing trajectory.

Additional future research efforts should seek to expand our understanding of the various populations for which tailoring of computer-based interventions may be critical and the specific-person characteristics on which to tailor. These data will inform us how to best develop interventions that can optimally benefit from a computer's ability to readily provide varying interventions that depend on individual characteristics to increase the efficacy of a computer-based intervention for various subpopulations. Moreover, additional research on how to best use technology to provide "in vivo" interventions to youth may further enhance the efficacy of such tools. This research may include providing multimedia text messaging and text messaging delivered via cell phones, as well as video and audio delivered to iPods and other portable devices to provide effective prevention messages in any setting.

Overall, adoption of such empirically supported technology may play a critical role in improving community-based substance abuse prevention and treatment for youth in a manner that enables rapid diffusion and widespread adoption of science-based interventions.

REFERENCES

1. Monitoring the Future: a continuing study of American youth. Available at: www.monitoringthefuture.org. Accessed May 15, 2007
2. Bollinger LC, Bush C, Califano JA, et al. *Under the Counter: The Diversion and Abuse of Controlled Prescription Drugs in the U.S.* New York, NY: National Center on Addiction and Substance Abuse at Columbia University; 2005
3. Partnership for a Drug-Free America. The Partnership Attitude Tracking Study: teens in grades 7 through 12. Available at: www.rwjf.org/research/researchdetail.jsp?id=2722&ia=131. Accessed January 31, 2007
4. King KM, Chassin L. A prospective study of the effects of age of initiation of alcohol and drug use on young adult substance dependence. *J Stud Alcohol Drugs.* 2007;68:256–265
5. King KM, Meehan BT, Trim RS, Chassin L. Marker or mediator? The effects of adolescent substance use on young adult educational attainment. *Addiction.* 2006;101:1730–1740
6. Mathers M, Toumbourou JW, Catalano RF, Williams J, Patton GC. Consequences of youth tobacco use: a review of prospective behavioral studies. *Addiction.* 2006;101:948–958
7. Hopfer CJ, Mikulich SK, Crowley TJ. Heroin use among adolescents in treatment for substance use disorders. *J Am Acad Child Adolesc Psychiatry.* 2000;39:1316–1323
8. Lee LM, Fleming PL. Trends in human immunodeficiency virus diagnoses among women in the United States, 1994–1998. *J Am Med Womens Assoc.* 2001;56:94–99
9. Faggiano F, Vigna-Taglianti FD, Versino E, Zambon A, Borraccino A, Lemma P. School-based prevention for illicit drugs' use. *Cochrane Database Syst Rev.* 2005;(2):CD003020

10. National Institute on Drug Abuse. Preventing drug use among children and adolescents. NIH publication 04-4112(b). Available at: www.drugabuse.gov/Prevention/Prevopen.html. Accessed January 31, 2007

11. Substance Abuse and Mental Health Services Administration. TIP 32: treatment of adolescents with substance use disorders. DHHS publication 99-3283. Available at: www.ncbi.nlm.nih.gov/books/bv.fcgi?highlight=treatment,tip,adolescents&rid=hstat5.chapter.56031. Accessed May 23, 2007

12. Skiba D, Monroe J, Wodarski JS. Adolescent substance use: reviewing the effectiveness of preventing strategies. *Soc Work.* 2004;49:343–353

13. Bickel WK, Marsch LA. A future for drug abuse prevention and treatment in the 21st century: applications of computer-based information technologies. In: Henningfield J, Bickel WK, eds. *Substance Abuse in the 21st Century.* Baltimore, MD: Johns Hopkins Press; 2007:35–43

14. Bickel WK, McLellan AT. Can management by outcome invigorate substance abuse treatment? Microincentives and the quality of care. *Am J Addict.* 1996;5:281–291

15. Ennett ST, Ringwalt CL, Thorne J, et al. A comparison of current practice in school-based substance use prevention programs with meta-analysis findings. *Prev Sci.* 2003;4:1–14

16. McLellan AT, Carise D, Kleber HD. Can the national addiction treatment infrastructure support the public's demand for quality care? *J Subst Abuse Treat.* 2003;25:117–121

17. Fox S. Pew Internet & American Life Project: prescription drugs online—one in four Americans have looked online for drug information, but few have ventured into the online drug marketplace. Available at: www.pewinternet.org/pdfs/PIP_Prescription_Drugs_Online.pdf. Accessed May 15, 2007

18. Market Data Retrieval. *Technology in Education 2001.* Shelton, CT: Market Data Retrieval; 2001

19. McKinsey & Co. *Connecting K-12 Schools to the Information Superhighway.* New York, NY: McKinsey & Co; 1995

20. Roker D, Coleman J. Education and advice about illegal drugs: what do young people want? *Drugs Educ Prev Policy.* 1997;4:53–64

21. Cook DA. Learning and cognitive styles in Web-based learning: theory, evidence, and application. *Acad Med.* 2005;80:266–278

22. Cook DA, Thompson WG, Thomas KG, Thomas MR, Pankratz VS. Impact of self-assessment questions and learning styles in Web-based learning: a randomized, controlled, crossover trial. *Acad Med.* 2006;81:231–238

23. Orlandi MA, Dozier CE, Marta MA. Computer-assisted strategies for substance abuse prevention: opportunities and barriers. *J Consult Clin Psychol.* 1990;58:425–431

24. Pagliaro LA. The history and development of CAI: 1926–1981. *Alberta J Educ Res.* 1983;29: 75–84

25. Binder C. Behavioral fluency: a new paradigm. *Educ Technol.* 1993;33:8–14

26. Binder C. Behavioral fluency: evolution of a new paradigm. *Behav Anal.* 1996;19:163–197

27. Dougherty KM, Johnson JM. Overlearning, fluency, and automaticity. *Behav Anal.* 1996;19: 289–292

28. Lieberman DC, Lynn MC. Learning to learn revisited: computers and the development of self directed skills. *J Res Comput Educ.* 1991;231:373–395

29. Marsch LA, Bickel WK. The efficacy of computer-based HIV/AIDS education for injection drug users. *Am J Health Behav.* 2004;28:316–327

30. Marsch LA, Bickel WK, Grabinski MJ, Badger GJ. Applying computer technology to substance abuse prevention science: results of a preliminary examination. *J Child Adolesc Subst Abuse.* 2007;16:69–94

31. Streufert S, Swezey R. Simulation and related research methods in environmental psychology. In: Singer J, Baum A, eds. *Advances in Environmental Psychology.* 1985:99–117

32. Gustafson DH, Bosworth K, Chewning B, Hawkins RP. Computer-based health promotion: combining technological advances with problem-solving techniques to effect successful health behavior changes. *Annu Rev Public Health.* 1987;8:387–415

33. Johnson KR, Layng TV. Breaking the structuralist barrier: literacy and numeracy with fluency. *Am Psychol.* 1992;47:1475–1490

34. Kommers PAM, Grabinger S, Dunlap JC. *Hypermedia Learning Environments: Instructional Design and Integration.* Mahwah, NJ: Lawrence Erlbaum; 1996

35. Kozma RB. Learning with media. *Rev Educ Res.* 1991;61:179–211

36. Rimal RN, Flora JA. Interactive technology attributes in health promotion: practical and theoretical issues. In: Street RL, Gold WR, Manning T, eds. *Health Promotion and Interactive Technology: Theoretical Applications and Future Directions.* Mahwah, NJ: Lawrence Erlbaum; 1997:19–38

37. Botvin GJ, Baker E, Dusenbury L, Botivn EM, Diaz T. Long-term follow-up results of a randomized drug abuse prevention trial in a white middle-class population. *JAMA.* 1995;273:1106–1112

38. Botvin GJ, Epstein JA, Baker E, Diaz T, Ifill-Williams M. School-based drug abuse prevention with inner-city minority youth. In: Botvin GJ, Schinke S, eds. *The Etiology and Prevention of Drug Abuse Among Minority Youth.* New York, NY: Haworth Press; 1997

39. Callas P, Flynn BS, Worden JK. *Psychosocial Factors Associated With Alcohol Use Among Early Adolescents.* Working paper. Burlington, VT: Office of Health Promotion Research, College of Medicine, University of Vermont; 1999

40. Costa FM, Jessor R, Turbin MS. Transition into adolescent problem drinking: the role of psychosocial risk and protective factors. *J Stud Alcohol.* 1999;60:480–490

41. Flay BR, Petraitis J, Hu FB. Psychosocial risk and protective factors for adolescent tobacco use. *Nicotine Tob Res.* 1999;1(suppl 1):S59–S65

42. Malow RM, Dévieux JG, Jennings T, Lucenko BA, Kalichman SC. Substance-abusing adolescents at varying levels of HIV risk: psychosocial characteristics, drug use, and sexual behavior. *J Subst Abuse.* 2001;13:103–117

43. D'Angelo L, DiClemente R. Sexually transmitted diseases including human immunodeficiency virus infection. In: DiClemente RJ, Hansen WB, Ponton LE, eds. *Handbook of Adolescent Health Risk Behavior.* New York, NY: Plenum; 1996:333–367

44. Millstein SG, Moscicki AB. Sexually transmitted disease in female adolescents: effects of psychosocial factors and high risk behaviors. *J Adolesc Health.* 1995;17:83–90

45. Rotheram-Borus MJ. Expanding the range of interventions to reduce HIV among adolescents. *AIDS.* 2000;14(suppl 1):S33–S40

46. Langer LM, Tubman JG. Risky sexual behavior among substance-abusing adolescents: psychosocial and contextual factors. *Am J Orthopsychiatry.* 1997;67:315–322

47. Siegal HA, Li L, Leviton LC, et al. Under the influence: risky sexual behavior and substance abuse among driving under the influence offenders. *Sex Transm Dis.* 1999;26:87–92

48. Rotheram-Borus MJ, Mann T, Chabon B. Amphetamine use and its correlates among youths living with HIV. *AIDS Educ Prev.* 1999;11:232–242

49. Shoptaw S, Reback CJ, Frosch DL, Rawson RA. Stimulant abuse treatment as HIV prevention. *J Addict Dis.* 1998;17:19–32

50. Doherty MC, Garfein RS, Monterroso E, Brown D, Vlahov D. Correlates of HIV infection among young adult short-term injection drug users. *AIDS.* 2000;14:717–726

51. Flom PL, Friedman SR, Kottiri BJ, et al. Stigmatized drug use, sexual partner concurrency, and other sex risk network and behavior characteristics of 18- to 24-year-old youth in a high-risk neighborhood. *Sex Transm Dis.* 2001;28:598–607

52. Holtzman D, Anderson JE, Kann L. HIV instruction, HIV knowledge, and drug injection among high school students in the United States. *Am J Public Health.* 1991;81:1596–1601

Adolesc Med 18 (2007) 357–369

Engaging Youth in E-Health Promotion: Lessons Learned From a Decade of TeenNet Research

Cameron D. Norman, PhD[a],

Harvey A. Skinner, PhD, CPsych[b],*

[a]Department of Public Health Sciences, University of Toronto, 155 College Street, Room 586, Toronto, Ontario, Canada M5T 3M7

[b]Faculty of Health, York University, 4700 Keele Street, Toronto, Ontario, Canada M3J 1P3

Cigarette smoking is a habit that, in North America, is initiated almost exclusively during youth (12–24 years of age) and, despite tremendous effort from public health agencies, remains a significant health problem facing adolescents and young adults.[1,2] This problem is exacerbated by a dearth of evidence-based programs that capture the interest of youth, are widely accessible, and respond to both the prevention and cessation needs of young people.[3] Web-assisted tobacco interventions (WATIs) may provide such an option to media-oriented, highly connected populations such as youth in Canada and the United States[4,5] who frequently use information and communication technology (ICT) as a source of health information[4,6–9] and for building and maintaining social networks.[10]

The World Health Organization recommends that adolescent-oriented health information be interactive, involve active promotion, and use tailoring to meet the needs of individual adolescents while simultaneously having the ability to reach large numbers of them.[11] Networked tools such as the Internet provide the best opportunity to achieve all of these goals in ways that were previously unimaginable. Information technologies allow public health programs to connect with youth as they connect with each other. This new approach to delivering health information and programming is part of a larger set of technologies and strategies called e-health.[12]

Using ICT for health promotion, or behavioral e-health (cf, ref 13), has been successful at delivering effective behavior-change interventions.[14–18] Given the Internet's reach and availability, even small changes attributed to a behavioral

---

*Corresponding author.

E-mail address: harvey.skinner@yorku.ca (H. A. Skinner).

e-health intervention can translate into a large population health effect. Tobacco control is a leading area of behavioral e-health research[13,19–21] despite the challenges in applying standard research models to electronic smoking-cessation programs.[22,23] WATIs are a class of ICT interventions that have become popular because of their ease of proliferation, scalability, and relatively low cost compared with many other traditional forms of tobacco-control initiatives. Web-assisted behavior-change tools, in general, have achieved success in facilitating behavior change across a variety of health conditions,[15,17,24] with tobacco control being among the most widely studied and promising.[16,18–31]

Adolescent smoking remains a public health problem despite recent reductions in the overall cigarette-smoking rates within the population. In Canada, 16% of adolescents aged 15 to 19 smoke, and 9% smoke daily.[1] For young adults aged 20 to 24, this number jumps to 25%, the highest rate within the general population.[1,32] This suggests that a combined effort to prevent smoking uptake and support cessation must be maintained throughout adolescence to reduce the burden of smoking-related diseases on a population level now and in the future. WATI is a natural option to explore.

BACKGROUND

TeenNet Research was founded in 1995 with the aim of harnessing the potential of emerging ICTs to engage youth in health promotion.[33,34] Authentic youth engagement is achieved through a set of 5 guiding principles that inform each TeenNet project:
- participation (youth involved in all stages of development and delivery);
- relevance (focused on personal, social, and health issues identified by youth);
- autonomy (support and respect for individual choice);
- active (learning and fun); and
- access (addressing both absolute access and quality of access[35] while fostering the e-health literacy skills[36] required to fully use ICTs for health).

This approach is informed not only by multiple health behavior–change theories but also by the work of Friere and his critical pedagogy.[37,38] With his community-engagement approach, Friere argues that listening precedes dialogue, which then precedes action and suggests that only through authentic dialogue in which all parties have equitable voices can true informed action take place. From a practice standpoint, this means involving youth in creating leadership opportunities throughout the project and focusing on strengthening youth-adult partnerships.[39–42] This approach also expands focus beyond youth to include adults and organizations that work with youth. A multilevel approach places attention on supporting more than just individual change (eg, smoking cessation);

it should also focus on actions that transform organizations,[43] strengthen communities,[44,45] and promote system-level change.[46,47] It is embodied into a model called the Likelihood of Action Index (LAI), developed by Skinner[43] and Norman.[13] Collins and Ellickson[48] demonstrated the utility of taking an integrated, multitheory approach to health behavior change in their study of smoking initiation by adolescents in 10th grade. They found that logically combining different theories into a single model was superior to the individual models alone at predicting cigarette use 3 years later.

Although theories help explain and guide program content, they do not provide a means to put knowledge into action. To guide this process, TeenNet developed a series of models that would reflect its values and enable it to transform ideas into actionable outcomes. One of these models is called EIPARS; it represents the overall approach to engagement with youth.

EIPARS Model

TeenNet's engagement approach is captured in the 6-step EIPARS model for sustainable action with youth (Fig 1):
- engage (interested youth are connected and motivated to work in a peer relationship on an action project in their community);
- identify (youth explore their community and identify issues that concern them);
- plan (youth choose 1 issue and develop a strategy to address it);
- act (youth implement the project according to the plan the group developed);

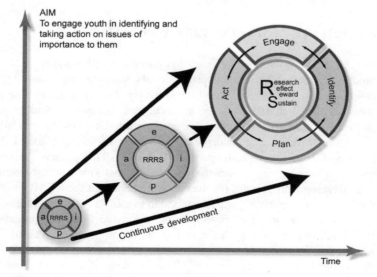

Fig 1 EIPARS 6-phase model.

- research, reflect, and reward (youth evaluate the effectiveness of the action project and reflect on the outcomes of the group processes); and
- sustain (ways to sustain the group and its action are considered; this stage is both independent and integrated throughout the model).

The EIPARS model has been used successfully with diverse youth groups in Canada and internationally.[49,50] Workbooks including process guides and tools for each step are available online at: www.globalyouthvoices.org/resources.html.

WATIs for Youth

Through the use of the EIPARS model, an interactive tool was developed with youth that met their needs and interest in reducing and eliminating cigarette use. The initial product to emerge from this process was CyberIsle (www.cyberisle.org), a virtual teens-only island that provides tools and information on social and health issues, particularly smoking. The site was developed in 1995 at a time when there were few adolescent health resources online and a global Web population of only 18 000 sites (compared with the >100 million in existence currently).[51] While completing the Web site, users are asked to input how many cigarettes they typically consume in a month (or would consider consuming if they became a smoker), and from this, a tailored Web experience leads them through the perceived benefits and actual consequences of smoking while aiding them in making plans to change.[52] This approach to screening and providing tailored content was used in the development of future programs as the site evolved over time and eventually spawned the Smoking Zine Web site.

CASE STUDY: THE SMOKING ZINE WEB SITE

Although CyberIsle provides a holistic environment for discussing tobacco use, stakeholders (youth, teachers, health professionals) have expressed desire to have a cessation-and-prevention tool that is exclusively dedicated to smoking. This would enable the Web site to serve as a curriculum resource and provide a more-focused option for smokers who are interested in cessation. Using an iterative design process that incorporates elements of usability and EIPARS called the Spiral Technology Action Research (STAR) approach,[53] CyberIsle was refined in various stages over the years and transformed into the Smoking Zine. The development process for the Smoking Zine and the STAR model are described in detail elsewhere[53] and illustrated in Fig 2. The new program adopted a "street-wise" look and feel based on an extensive feedback process that involved youth drawn from both urban and rural communities. The usability-testing process ensures that the intervention is accessible and functions as designed under evaluation conditions.[54] The Smoking Zine is completed in 5 distinct stages, which are described in detail in Table 1.

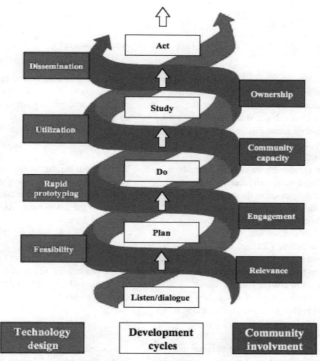

Fig 2 STAR model. (Reproduced with permission from Skinner HA, Maley O, Norman CD. *Health Promot Pract.* 2006;7:408.)

From 2000 to 2003, TeenNet undertook a series of evaluations of the Smoking Zine in settings that ranged from libraries to health centers, urban and rural, including 2 randomized trials. The first evaluation involved 118 youth ($N = 65$ girls) and 16 different locations throughout the province of Ontario, Canada. All participants were randomly assigned to either complete the Smoking Zine or a control condition (a structured search task on the Web). The results of the trial suggested that it was possible to conduct a randomized trial in a naturalistic setting using a Web-based tool. The small sample size did not permit reliable analyses of impact in statistical terms; however, when the measured response was compared with qualitative feedback provided from the surveys, the results encouraged pursuit of a larger trial.

Evaluation

In 2001, TeenNet began collaborations with the 2 main school boards in Toronto, Ontario, and Toronto Public Health to address the need for programming that supported prevention, cessation, and the school curriculum. Building on the results of the pilot evaluation, the Smoking Zine was further redesigned with

Table 1
The Smoking Zine stages

Smoking Zine Stage	Process/Concept
"Makin' Cents"	
Participants input the number of cigarette packs they smoke (or would smoke if they were to start) in 1 month. The market value of the cigarette packs is calculated into an annual total. Participants then spend this amount in a virtual shopping mall.	This stage was designed to raise consciousness of the cost of cigarette purchases relative to other consumer goods.
"It's Your Life"	
Participants complete a short assessment about their smoking behavior (frequency, amount smoked), which serves as the basis for the program's tailoring. Tailoring is based on whether someone is a smoker, nonsmoker, or an experimental/social smoker.	This stage is an assessment of smoking status and provides personalized feedback on the level of relative risk based on the results of the assessment. Awareness could be added here.
"To Change or Not to Change"	
This quiz is tailored to the user's smoking status (identified in step 2) and allows them to assess their readiness to change (quit or reduce smoking). In addition, youth assess how important this change is and their confidence in being able to change.	This component assesses (1) readiness (stage of change), (2) confidence (self-efficacy), and (3) importance (self-determination).
"It's Your Decision"	
This section creates a decision balance that displays the pros and cons related to smoking and being smoke free. After completion of the matrix, users can clearly see their thoughts about smoking and reasons to quit or reduce their tobacco consumption or stay at their current level.	This stage examines the pros and cons of being a nonsmoker versus a smoker (decision balance). A decision balance helps advance user's readiness to change.
"What Now?"	
This section brings together results from the previous stages in an easy-to-use and comprehensive format. For smokers who are ready to quit, the Smoking Zine will guide them in creating a personalized quit program. If the participant is not ready to quit, then the Smoking Zine will take them to a personal forecast quiz. The quiz examines other areas of the person's life that may relate to their smoking behavior, such as close relationships and availability of social support.	Identification of readiness, barriers, and assets are core components for a successful change plan. This stage helps develop a quit plan that includes a specific date, method of cessation, support mechanisms, relapse-prevention strategies, and outcome rewards (cognitive/behavioral change plan).

feedback from school officials and youth, and a more extensive randomized trial was designed and implemented over the following 2 years.

In 2003, a 2-group randomized, controlled trial was implemented with 1402 male and female students in grades 9 to 11 from 14 secondary schools in Toronto

(C.D.N., O. Maley, X. Li, and H.A.S., unpublished data, 2007),[22] with 211 (15%) assessed as smokers at baseline. Eighty-one classes were sampled from 14 secondary schools in the greater Toronto area, one of the most multicultural cities in the world. Thirty-nine percent of the students were in 9th grade ($n = 548$), 30% in 10th grade ($n = 418$), and 31% in 11th grade ($n = 436$). Participants completed either the Smoking Zine or another interactive exercise on the Internet that was designed to promote critical thinking and skill development in using online health information or e-health literacy.[36] The Web-site experience was supplemented by a group discussion based on motivational interviewing,[55] followed by tailored e-mails that included brief motivational messages that were sent over the course of 6 months. Resistance to smoking, behavioral intentions to smoke, and cigarette consumption were assessed at baseline, posttest, and postintervention at 3- and 6-month follow-ups by using a multilevel modeling process,[56,57] which facilitated analysis of change at the individual, class, and grade levels.

The trial was the largest of its kind and illustrated both the challenges and opportunities inherent in school-based e-health research, from recruitment to delivery of a program designed around an intervention that has a Web site as its core component. Outcomes were assessed by using a longitudinal multilevel modeling approach that compared baseline scores on the 3 dependent variables over time. Although no statistical main effects were detected, several cross-level interactions pointed to specific areas in which the program was effective. A detailed outline of the procedures, methodology, and discussion of the finding is available elsewhere (C.D.N., O. Maley, X. Li, and H.A.S., unpublished data, 2007). In general, the program had a greater effect with nonsmokers than smokers, likely due in part to the challenge of changing a complex health behavior in a single session.

Key Results

Baseline health-risk factors were significantly higher for smokers than nonsmokers and included alcohol use (number of days used and number of days on which >5 drinks were consumed), drug use, anxiety, perceived stress, and satisfaction with relationships. Results of an independent-samples t test between smokers and nonsmokers on the overall risk scale supported that smokers engaged in more high-risk behaviors ($P <. 001$).

The intervention had the greatest influence on boys, both increasing resistance to smoking at 3 months and decreasing intentions to smoke from baseline to 6 months. The already-low levels of actual cigarette use were also decreased at 3 months. For girls, resistance increased at 3 months, and both 9th- and 10th-grade girls decreased their intentions to smoke at 3 months. However, no impact was detected on cigarette use. These findings suggest that girls may require additional supports or that modification is necessary to have a greater influence in preventing smoking. There were 3 core outcomes of interest among nonsmokers.

Resistance to Smoking Initiation

No overall effect was detected on resistance to smoking attributable to the Smoking Zine, although a significant cross-level interaction was detected for 10th-grade students at the 3-month follow-up. However, the absence of immediate impact at posttest adds uncertainty as to whether the change was attributed to the intervention or some other factor.

Behavioral Intentions

No significant main effect of group was detected. However, significant interaction effects were detected among specific subgroups. During the model-development process, most of the variance was accounted for at the individual level, with only modest influences of grade. No significant effect of gender was detected; however, a significant interaction of gender and group was detected. The final model was assessed by examining intraclass interactions. Two significant interactions were found for 9th- and 11th-grade boys and 10th-graders overall. Thus, these 3 subpopulations showed a statistically significant ($P < .05$) increase in intentions not to smoke that were attributed to the Smoking Zine at the immediate posttest. Importantly, these effects were maintained at the 3- and 6-month follow-ups for each interaction.

Cigarette Use

We compared cigarette use at baseline with use at the 6-month follow-up. Consistent with our other analyses, no effect was found for school or class, with only a small effect of grade. Therefore, individual-level random parameters were retained in all statistical models. An interaction effect was detected when baseline standardized scores of resistance, intention and cigarette use, group assignment, and gender were modeled.

In summary, both nonsmoking boys and girls significantly increased their resistance to smoking initiation at the 3-month follow-up, whereas boys in all grades and 10-grade girls decreased their intentions to smoke through the 6-month follow-up. Cigarette use was also reduced at 3 months for boys in all grades. No significant difference in smoking-related outcomes was detected between groups with smokers, although cigarette use decreased significantly for both groups at the 6-month follow-up.

DISCUSSION

Our evaluation of the Smoking Zine, when integrated into the classroom conditions, can be an effective tool for smoking prevention for specific groups. We found that smokers require more time to fully use the program, because many smokers did not complete the entire 5-stage program. The reason for this lay in the architecture of stage 5, which helps smokers recognize triggers for smoking, anticipate situational barriers to quitting, identify supports, and build a quit plan if they indicate they are interested in quitting earlier in stage 3. Conversely, nonsmokers and smokers who are not interested in quitting have far fewer activities and are more likely to finish.

Teachers and school administrators were unanimous in their approval of the Smoking Zine resource, and each school had expressed interest in doing additional work with the program in future projects. As a result, TeenNet began working with teachers and other partners to explore ways of integrating the Smoking Zine more fully into a system that reflected the differences in classroom environments and available resources. The result was the Virtual Classroom on Tobacco Control (VCTC; www.takingitglobal.org/tiged/projects/tobacco), co-created with the Ontario Physical and Health Education Association and TakingITGlobal (www.takingitglobal.org), a youth-serving organization that promotes global social engagement via the Internet. The VCTC includes downloadable activity plans and fact sheets for students, and it allows teachers to link to each other to share ideas and permits their classes to link together to facilitate learning across geographical distances. Part of the program is a 7-chapter program guide for teachers that provides background information, references, and lesson plans that include strategies for incorporating the Smoking Zine and VCTC into classes of different sizes, compositions, and lengths. All of these tools are available for download at www.youthvoices.ca, which enables classrooms around the world to benefit from this program.

CONCLUSIONS

The opportunities to engage youth globally in health promotion has only increased with the advent of Web 2.0 technologies[58] such as wikis[59] (easily edited Web pages), blogs[60] (online diaries), and social-networking sites such as MySpace[61] and Facebook.[62] These new technologies not only enable youth to create content without having knowledge of computer programming, but they also provide new ways to establish or grow social networks. More than half (55%) of US adolescents aged 12 to 17 report using social-networking sites, with 48% visiting them daily or more and 22% visiting multiple times each day.[10] Even mainstream medicine is considering the benefits of tools that enable dynamic, democratic, social interactions using Web 2.0 technologies for transforming health care.[63,64] Another prominent area for exploration is mobile phone technology as cameras, Web browsers, mp3 players, and video text-messaging capabilities become standard features on handheld devices that increasingly blur the distinction between telephone, computer, and home entertainment system. WATIs delivered through mobile phones have already shown promise in randomized trials with young people and adults alike[65] and will increase in sophistication over time.

Although technology will inevitably change, so too will the way that current technologies are used. Where WATIs were once designed as stand-alone tools, the future is likely to see these online programs become integrated within offline activities. Just as TeenNet has sought to create virtual classrooms that bridge online and physical learning environments, so too will WATIs begin to more tightly integrate with adolescent health clinics, community groups, and other health service providers. This integration will build on the strengths of ICT in conducting assessments, providing information, and connecting youth globally with the relationship-building and security strengths that face-to-face encounters offer. It is not hard to envision a scenario in the near future where assessments performed on a mobile phone are used to assist a health provider in designing a cessation strategy that incorporates an interactive Web site and is supported by downloadable video motivational messages with links to an online social network of people who are trying to quit smoking. Last, it is increasingly likely that tobacco control will continue to go global in scope and that ICT will play an increasing role in facilitating cessation, prevention, and policy changes to support adolescent health on a worldwide basis.

TeenNet has linked youth in Canada with those in Africa to identify common areas of concern around both local and global health issues as well as engaging youth across the Middle East in health promotion using the EIPARS process.[50] These examples illustrate the impact and importance of bridging cultural and geopolitical boundaries through ICT-youth engagement. The ratification of the World Health Organization Framework Convention on Tobacco Control[66] has placed a greater demand for knowledge and "lessons learned" that youth are already eager to provide if we listen to them. TeenNet has responded to some of these challenges by culturally translating the Smoking Zine into Hebrew, Arabic, French, and both simplified and Mandarin Chinese, creating new versions of the Web site for different groups that are relevant to contexts beyond North America. As the tobacco industry focuses on "emerging" or "dark markets" in both the developed and developing worlds,[67] the need to link tobacco-control expertise internationally is critical.

ACKNOWLEDGMENTS

We acknowledge the current and past leadership with TeenNet Research (Meg Morrison, Oonagh Maley, Charlotte Lombardo, Sherry Biscope, Sarah Flicker, Andrea Ridgley, Malcolm Koo, Jill Charnaw-Burger, and Suhail Abualsameed); Dr Xiaoqiang Li for assistance with data analysis on the Smoking Zine trial; and the hundreds of youth and adult advisors who contributed ideas and energy toward promoting health with us since 1995.

REFERENCES

1. Health Canada. Canadian Tobacco Use Monitoring Survey. Available at: www.hc-sc.gc.ca/hl-vs/tobac-tabac/research-recherche/stat/ctums-esutc/index_e.html. Accessed May 25, 2007

2. National Cancer Institute. *Changing Adolescent Smoking Prevalence: Where It Is and Why.* Bethesda, MD: US Department of Health and Human Services, National Institutes of Health, National Cancer Institute; 2001

3. Bader P, Skinner HA. *Use of Technology for Youth Smoking Prevention and Cessation.* Ottawa, Ontario, Canada: Health Canada; 2003

4. Environics Research Group. *Young Canadians in a Wired World: What Are Youth Doing Online, and What Do Their Parents Need to Know?* Toronto, Ontario, Canada: Environics Research Group; 2001. Report pn4737

5. Lenhart A, Madden M, Hitlin P. Pew Internet & American Life Project: teens and technology—youth are leading the transition to a fully wired and mobile nation. Available at: www.pewinternet.org/pdfs/PIP_Teens_Tech_July2005web.pdf. Accessed July 11, 2007

6. Hanson DL, Derry HA, Resnick PJ, Richardson CR. Adolescents searching for health information on the internet: an observational study. *J Med Internet Res.* 2003;5:e25. Available at: www.jmir.org/2003/4/e25

7. Gray NJ, Klein JD, Cantrill JA, Noyce PR. Adolescent girls' use of the Internet for health information: issues beyond access. *J Med Syst.* 2002;26:545–553

8. Rideout V. *Generation rx.com: How Young People Use the Internet for Health Information.* Washington, DC: Henry J. Kaiser Family Foundation; 2001

9. Borzekowski DL, Rickert VI. Adolescent cybersurfing for health information: a new resource that crosses barriers. *Arch Pediatr Adolesc Med.* 2001;155:813–817

10. Lenhart A, Madden. Social networking Web sites and teens: an overview. Pew Internet Project Data Memo. Available at: www.pewinternet.org/pdfs/PIP_SNS_Data_Memo_Jan_2007.pdf. Accessed July 11, 2007

11. World Health Organization/United Nations Population Fund/United Nations Children's Fund Study Group on Programming for Adolescent Health. *Programming for Adolescent Health and Development: Report of a WHO/UNFPA/UNICEF Study Group on Programming for Adolescent Health.* Saillon, Switzerland: World Health Organization; 1999. Report 886

12. Eysenbach G. What is e-health? *J Med Internet Res.* 2001;3:e20. Available at: www.jmir.org/2001/2/e20/

13. Norman CD. *The Web of Influence: Evaluating the Impact of Internet Interventions on Adolescent Smoking Cessation and eHealth Literacy* [dissertation]. Toronto, Ontario, Canada: University of Toronto; 2005

14. Christensen H, Griffiths KM, Korten A. Web-based cognitive behavior therapy: analysis of site usage and changes in depression and anxiety scores. *J Med Internet Res.* 2002;4:e3. Available at: www.jmir.org/2002/1/e3

15. Evers KE, Prochaska JM, Prochaska JO, Driskell M, Cummins CO, Velicer WF. Strengths and weaknesses of health behavior change programs on the Internet. *J Health Psychol.* 2003;8:63–70

16. Norman CD, Skinner HA. *Internet-Based Behavior Change: A Systematic Review.* Toronto, Ontario, Canada: University of Toronto; 2004

17. Ritterband LM, Gonder-Frederick LA, Cox DJ, Clifton AD, West RW, Borowitz SM. Internet interventions: in review, in use, and into the future. *Prof Psychol Res Pr.* 2003;34:527–534

18. Griffiths F, Lindenmeyer A, Powell J, Lowe P, Thorogood M. Why are health care interventions delivered over the Internet? A systematic review of the published literature. *J Med Internet Res.* 2006;8:e10. Available at: www.jmir.org/2006/2/e10

19. Etter JF. Comparting the efficacy of two Internet-based, computer tailored smoking cessation programs: a randomized trial. *J Med Internet Res.* 2005;7:e2. Available at: www.jmir.org/2005/1/e2

20. Etter JF, le Houezec J, Landfeldt B. Impact of messages on concomitant use of nicotine replacement therapy and cigarettes: a randomized trial on the Internet. *Addiction.* 2003;98:941–950

21. Feil EG, Noell J, Lichtenstein E, Boles SM, McKay HG. Evaluation of an Internet-based smoking cessation program: lessons learned from a pilot study. *Nicotine Tob Res.* 2003;5:189–194

22. Feil EG. Response to CATCH-IT report by Cameron Norman: Evaluation of an Internet-based smoking cessation program: Lessons learned from a pilot study. *J Med Internet Res.* 2004;6:e48. Available at: www.jmir.org/2004/4/e48

23. Norman CD. CATCH-IT report: evaluation of an Internet-based smoking cessation program: lessons learned from a pilot study. *J Med Internet Res.* 2005;6:e47; discussion e48. Available at: www.jmir.org/2004/4/e47

24. Christensen H, Griffiths KM, Jorm AF. Delivering interventions for depression by using the Internet: randomised controlled. *BMJ.* 2004;328:265

25. Malone RE, Bero LA. Cigars, youth, and the Internet link. *Am J Public Health.* 2000;90(5): 790–792

26. Woodruff SI, Edwards CC, Conway TL, Elliott SP. Pilot test of an Internet virtual world chat room for rural teen smokers. *J Adolesc Health.* 2001;29:239–243

27. Lenert L, Munoz RF, Stoddard J, et al. Design and pilot evaluation of an Internet smoking cessation program. *J Am Med Inform Assoc.* 2003;10:16–20

28. Bock BC, Graham AL, Sciamanna CN, et al. Smoking cessation treatment on the Internet: content, quality, and usability. *Nicotine Tob Res.* 2004;6:207–219

29. Eng TR. Emerging technologies for cancer prevention and other population health challenges. *J Med Internet Res.* 2005;7:e30. Available at: www.jmir.org/2005/3/e30

30. McClure JB, Greene SM, Wiese C, Johnson KE, Alexander G, Strecher VJ. Interest in an online smoking cessation program and effective recruitment strategies: results from Project Quit. *J Med Internet Res.* 2006;8:e14. Available at: www.jmir.org/2006/3/e14

31. Cobb KN, Graham LA. Characterizing Internet searchers of smoking cessation information. *J Med Internet Res.* 2006 19;8:e17. Available at: www.jmir.org/2006/3/e17

32. Bader P, Travis HE, Skinner HA. Knowledge synthesis of smoking cessation among employed and unemployed and unemployed young adults (18–24): the neglected population. *Am J Public Health.* 2007; In press

33. Skinner HA, Maley O, Smith L, Morrison M. New frontiers: using the Internet to engage teens in substance abuse prevention and treatment. In: Monte P, Colby S, eds. *Adolescence, Alcohol, and Substance Abuse: Reaching Teens Through Brief Interventions.* New York, NY: Guilford; 2001

34. Skinner HA, Morrison M, Bercovitz K, et al. Using the Internet to engage youth in health promotion. *Promot Educ.* 1997;4:23–25

35. Skinner HA, Biscope S, Poland B. Quality of Internet access: barrier behind Internet use statistics. *Soc Sci Med.* 2003;57:875–880

36. Norman CD, Skinner HA. eHealth literacy: essential skills for consumer health in a networked world. *J Med Internet Res.* 2006;8:e9. Available at: www.jmir.org/2006/2/e9

37. Freire P. *Education for Critical Consciousness.* New York, NY: Continuum; 1973

38. Freire P. *Pedagogy of the Oppressed.* New York, NY: Continuum; 1970

39. Camino LA. Youth-adult partnerships: entering new territory in community work and research. *Appl Dev Sci.* 2000;4(suppl 1):11–20

40. Ginwright S, James T. From assets to agents of change: social justice, organizing, and youth development. *New Dir Youth Dev.* 2002;96:27–46

41. Zeldin S. Youth as agents of adult and community development: mapping the process and outcomes of youth engaged in organizational governance. *Appl Dev Sci.* 2004;8:75–90

42. Zeldin S, Camino LA, Mook C. The adoption of innovation in youth organizations: creating the conditions for youth-adult partnerships. *J Community Psychol.* 2005;33:121–135

43. Skinner HA. *Promoting Health Through Organizational Change.* San Francisco, CA: Benjamin Cummings; 2002

44. Best A, Stokols D, Green LW, Leischow S, Holmes B, Buchholz K. An integrative framework for community partnering to translate theory into effective health promotion practice. *Am J Health Promot.* 2003;18:168–176

45. Kretzmann JP, McKnight JL. *Building Communities From the Inside Out: A Path Towards Finding and Mobilizing a Community's Assets.* Chicago, IL: ACTA; 1993

46. Best A, Trochim W, Moor G, et al. Systems thinking for knowledge integration: new models for policy-research collaboration. In: Casebeer A, Harrison A, Mark AE, eds. *Innovations in Health Care: A Reality Check.* London, United Kingdom: Palgrave MacMillan: 2007
47. Westley F, Zimmerman B, Patton M. *Getting to Maybe: How the World Is Changed.* Toronto, Ontario, Canada: Random House Canada; 2006
48. Collins RL, Ellickson PL. Integrating four theories of adolescent smoking. *Subst Use Misuse.* 2004;39:179–209
49. Bader R, Wanono R, Hamden S, Skinner HA. Global youth voices: engaging Bedouin youth in health promotion in the Middle East. *Can J Public Health.* 2007;98:21–25
50. Ridgley A, Maley O, Skinner HA. Youth voices: engaging youth in health promotion using media technologies. *Can Issues.* 2004;Fall:21–24
51. Walton M. Web reaches new milestone: 100 million sites. Available at: http://edition.cnn.com/2006/TECH/internet/11/01/100millionwebsites/index.html. Accessed January 23, 2007
52. Mills C, Stephens T, Wilkins K. Summary report of the Workshop on Data for Monitoring Tobacco Use [in English, French]. *Health Rep.* 1994;6:377–387
53. Skinner HA, Maley O, Norman CD. Developing Internet-based eHealth promotion programs: the Spiral Technology Action Research (STAR) model. *Health Promot Pract.* 2006;7:406–417
54. Baecker R, Buxton W. *Readings in Human-Computer Interaction: A Multi-disciplinary Approach.* San Mateo, CA: Kaufmann; 1987
55. Miller WR, Rollnick S. *Motivational Interviewing: Preparing People for Change.* 2nd ed. New York, NY: Guilford Press; 2002
56. Snijders TAB, Bosker RJ. *Multilevel Analysis: An Introduction to Basic and Advanced Multilevel Modeling.* London, United Kingdom: Sage; 1999
57. Hox JJ. *Applied Multilevel Analysis.* Amsterdam, Netherlands: TT-Publikaties; 1995
58. Wikipedia. Web 2.0. Available at: http://en.wikipedia.org/wiki/Web_2. Accessed September 23, 2006
59. Wikipedia. Wiki. Available at: http://en.wikipedia.org/wiki/Wiki. Accessed September 23, 2006
60. Wikipedia. Blog. Available at: http://en.wikipedia.org/wiki/Blog. Accessed September 23, 2006
61. MySpace. MySpace home page. Available at: www.myspace.com. Accessed September 23, 2006
62. Facebook. Facebook home page. Available at: www.facebook.com. Accessed July 11, 2007
63. Deshpande A, Jadad AR. Web 2.0: could it help move the health system into the 21st century. *J Mens Health Gender.* 2006;3:332–336
64. Giustini D. How Web 2.0 is changing medicine. *BMJ.* 2006;333:1283–1284
65 Rodgers A, Corbett T, Bramley D, et al. Do u smoke after txt? Results of a randomized trial of smoking cessation using mobile phone text messaging. *Tob Control.* 2005;14:255–261
66. World Health Organization. WHO framework convention on tobacco control. Available at: www.who.int/tobacco/framework/WHO_FCTC_english.pdf. Accessed May 28, 2007
67. Carter SM. Going below the line: creating transportable brands for Australia's dark market. *Tob Control.* 2003;12(suppl 3):iii87–iii94

Adolesc Med 18 (2007) 370–382

Adolescents, the Internet, and Health Literacy

Nicola J. Gray, PhD, MRPharmS*

Division for Social Research in Medicines and Health, School of Pharmacy, University of Nottingham, University Park, Nottingham NG7 2RD, England

Adolescents entering the adult world in the 21st century will read and write more than at any other time in human history. They will need advanced levels of literacy to perform their jobs, run their households, act as citizens, and conduct their personal lives. They will need literacy to cope with the flood of information they will find everywhere they turn.

International Reading Association[1]

Although discussion is rife, a review of the empirical work surrounding adolescent health literacy and adolescents' use of the Internet for health information shows that we still have much to explore.[2] The Institute of Medicine (IOM) report "Health Literacy: A Prescription to End Confusion"[3] crystallized the challenges that face global health services. For some time now, health literacy has been a topic for intense research and action for a relatively small number of academic and professional groups, but only recently has this topic been adopted as a priority for action by the broader health research and policy sectors. The statement from the International Reading Association cited above reinforces the urgency with which we need to equip our young people with literacy skills that will facilitate healthy and prosperous lives. These skills will include an ability to apply general literacy principles to specialized areas of their lives, including the complex and often unfamiliar terminology and concepts associated with health. This requires cooperation between health and education professionals, an investment in the future health of our population.

HEALTH LITERACY: DEFINITIONS, RESEARCH, AND POLICY

The operational definition of health literacy used in *Healthy People 2010*,[4] subsequently adopted by the IOM report, was "the degree to which individuals have the capacity to obtain, process and understand basic health information and services needed to make appropriate health decisions."[5] This is a broad definition

---

*Corresponding author.

E-mail address: nicola.gray@nottingham.ac.uk (N. J. Gray).

of health literacy, mirrored by others such as the World Health Organization.[6] Reflections on the World Health Organization definition of health literacy resulted in a tripartite model that describes skills other than functional health literacy and can be summarized as follows:

- functional literacy, to have the basic skills (reading and writing) to be able to function effectively in everyday situations;
- critical literacy, to critically analyze information and use this information to exert greater control over life events and situations; and
- interactive literacy, to extract information and derive meaning from different forms of communication and to apply new information to changing circumstances.[7]

These definitions go beyond reading and writing, yet much of the existing health literacy research relates to functional/basic literacy skills, primarily those of reading and comprehension.[8,9] Health literacy studies have sometimes used reading grade as a proxy measure; others have used scales such as the Rapid Estimate of Adult Literacy in Medicine (REALM).[10] When using REALM, individuals are asked to read aloud lists of medical terms that become more complex. Inevitably, more mistakes in pronunciation are made as the complexity increases, and that is how the test is scored.

Other approaches in this field include testing comprehension of the information within patient-education brochures and medication labels.[8] In contrast, very few studies have examined the "critical" or "interactive" aspects of health literacy that are integral to these definitions. These limitations are recognized in the IOM report. The IOM Committee on Health Literacy found that current tools could not explore differences in reading ability; lack of background knowledge in health-related domains, including biology; lack of familiarity with language; and cultural differences in approaches to health and health care.[3]

The American Medical Association has, for some years, led an ongoing campaign to improve health literacy.[11] Their concern is that people with the greatest health needs may have the least ability to read and comprehend health information. Adolescents are an important audience for all these initiatives. Unlike adults, who have few opportunities to come together to learn as a community, most adolescents in the developed world are in an educational infrastructure that provides opportunities for outreach. Their well-documented computer use and early adoption of new technology also suggest that online tools could be an effective means of increasing their health literacy skills for online and off-line use.

Health literacy should not be viewed as being dependent on the individual alone. There is a complex relationship between determinants of health and health literacy. For example, the Public Health Agency of Canada has a published list of determinants of health (Box 1).[12] The framework for Canada's program of

---

Box 1. Determinants of health: Public Health Agency of Canada[12]

- Income and social status
- Social support networks
- Education and literacy
- Employment/working conditions
- Social environments
- Physical environments
- Personal health practices and coping skills
- Healthy child development
- Biology and genetic endowment
- Health services
- Gender
- Culture

---

research into health literacy in 2003 showed that these determinants impact on health literacy[13]; it also showed actions that could address health literacy issues, including capacity development, community development, organizational development, and national policy. Improvements in skills will only be achieved by a range of initiatives working at both the individual and population level.

In September 2006, results of the first specific national assessment of health-literacy skills of America's adults (from the 2003 National Assessment of Adult Literacy [NAAL]) were published.[14] There was a battery of health literacy tasks compiled to test the skills of individuals aged ≥16 years. They tackled issues from 3 key aspects of health care: clinical, preventive, and navigation of the health system. The major demographic findings from the exercise are summarized in Box 2, including results indicating that most adults had intermediate health literacy, and that women and younger adults (aged <65 years) had higher health literacy than their counterparts.

There have been many studies conducted, mostly in the United States, to determine the consequences of inadequate health literacy. Many of these studies have found that poor health literacy has measurable negative effects on the patient's health and on the costs and utilization of health services that impact the whole population. These effects include lack of knowledge and skills; treatment failure and medication errors; increased risk of hospitalization; worse individual health outcomes; and higher health service costs.[15–20]

FOCUS ON ADOLESCENT HEALTH LITERACY

Most studies that have measured health literacy, its impact on health status, and use of health services have not included adolescents; the studies have mainly

---

Box 2. Findings from the health literacy tasks in the 2003 NAAL[14]

- The majority of the adults (53%) had intermediate health literacy (defined as "skills needed to perform moderately challenging literacy activities"), but 14% had "below basic" health literacy (defined as "no more than the most simple and concrete literacy skills").
- Women had higher average health literacy than men.
- White and Asian/Pacific Islander adults had higher average health literacy than those in other groups.
- Adults who spoke only English before school had higher average health literacy than those who spoke another language or >1 language including English.
- Younger adults (<65 y of age) had higher average health literacy than older adults.
- Average health literacy increased with higher educational attainment, starting with those who completed high school or obtained a general education diploma (GED).
- Those who were living below the poverty threshold had lower average health literacy than those in households above the threshold.

---

involved hospital patients, those with chronic conditions, and older adults.[8] One study that addressed the relationship between health literacy and gonorrhea-related care did include a wide cross-section of a US local population (aged 12–55 years),[21] but age-related differences were not examined in the analysis. We will see ongoing, inherited population health literacy challenges if the youngest members are not included in current initiatives.

The consequences of inadequate health literacy have great relevance for adolescents, although youth have not been a focus of previous health literacy research. For example, the incidence of treatment failure through noncompliance with medications is important in the context of birth control. If young women are not empowered and enabled to understand the instructions that come with their birth control pills, then unintended pregnancy is a very likely result. Similarly, if young people are not able to understand the risk factors for sexually transmitted infections such as HIV/AIDS or to follow basic instructions to protect themselves, then the incidence of these infections will continue their rapid rise in the adolescent population. Seemingly intractable adolescent health issues may have a root in inadequate health literacy.

The team who developed REALM for adults recently published their validation of the REALM-Teen tool with 1533 adolescents aged 10 to 19 years from Louisiana and North Carolina.[22] They concluded that REALM-Teen was valid and useful for assessing adolescent (functional) health literacy in the research or clinical setting. The average time to administer REALM-Teen was 3 minutes, which suggests that it might be feasible to administer in an office setting. It was possible to distinguish between 5 reading levels, from ≤3rd grade to ≥10th grade. The authors noted, however, that REALM-Teen could only detect low literacy (not specific grades) and was unable to diagnose reading or learning difficulties. REALM-Teen is also only available in English, because it is a word-recognition test that is unsuitable for phonetic languages such as Spanish.

The well-known Canadian health literacy research group, led by Irving Rootman at the University of Victoria, is undertaking a program of research regarding measurement of health literacy in schools.[23] Funded by the Canadian Institutes of Health Research until March 2008, they will develop and validate measures of health literacy that can respond to health needs in a school context. Barriers to effective health literacy programs in schools have included a lack of appropriate operational definition and assessment tools. The IOM report asserted that health education and literacy education are both essential to promoting health literacy in K-12 students, because the former provides health-related knowledge and the latter provides the skills for reading, writing, and comprehending text.[3]

With regard to health literacy in the online environment, a recent article by Norman and Skinner extends the discussion of health literacy definitions by introducing the concept of "e-health literacy" as "the ability to seek, find, understand, and appraise health information from electronic sources and apply the knowledge gained to addressing or solving a health problem."[24] They contend that e-health literacy is comprised of multiple literacies: traditional, health, information, scientific, media, and computer. Combining moderate skills across all 6 literacies, rather than needing mastery of any, gives online consumers the best chance to make the most of online health resources.

This concept of multiple literacies raises another interesting, yet often overlooked, aspect of health literacy. An individual may have high literacy in a certain area, such as a postgraduate with excellent general literacy, yet they could exhibit low health literacy. This might be because of a lack of experience with the health care system or specific difficulty with understanding medical terms. Conversely, an individual with a long-term medical condition, and great understanding of their medication, could have high health literacy but low general literacy. Similarly, someone with great Internet-use experience may find it easier to search for health information in this manner rather than try to negotiate our complex health care systems. Therefore, it is too simplistic to try and assume the level of an individual's health literacy as a parallel to their reading age.

Box 3. Examples of online challenges related to health literacy constructs[7]

Functional health literacy
- Spelling medical terms to put into search engines
- Understanding medical language used on health Web sites
- Constructing questions about health for use in e-mail or on Web sites

Critical health literacy
- Knowing whom to trust in the online environment (eg, when purchasing a product)
- Differentiating a large volume of information from different sources
- Looking for a second opinion (eg, cross-checking information from >1 Web site)

Interactive health literacy
- Acting on the online information (eg, not taking a performance enhancer)
- Using the information to start a conversation with a health professional
- Taking action to prevent a health problem (eg, monitoring pollen counts)

ADOLESCENTS' HEALTH INFORMATION–SEEKING BEHAVIOR AND USE OF THE INTERNET

Previous studies have shown that information about health and medicines is gathered over time from a complex network of personal and impersonal, lay and professional information sources.[25,26] One's ability to identify common symptoms and choose appropriate treatment strategies and evaluate their efficacy depends on personal "repertories" of health information. The Internet is a major health information source.[26] Health literacy skills determine the success with which information is processed. The factors that determine if new information is incorporated into an individual's repertory include the credibility of the information source and the saliency of the material to their own health concerns or those of a member of their social circle.

Recommendations from studies of adolescent Internet use have included the use of colloquial language for describing medical terms, construction of search strategies for commonly asked questions, and the creation of repositories of frequently asked questions.[27–31] These represent ways to help adolescents overcome challenges when searching for health information on the Internet. A study by my team sought to describe these challenges as a manifestation of their health-literacy skills[32]; different online searching problems were categorized by using the Nutbeam definition of health literacy[7] (Box 3). It concluded that the Internet could be a conduit to identify and remedy health-literacy deficits.

Other studies have identified such challenges without necessarily making the link explicit but nonetheless illuminating the issues. Hansen et al[33] observed adolescent searches for information related to preset tasks and found that their success varied. The greatest challenges were related to a task to find information about a local health service, but the sheer volume of possible sites retrieved by most search engines also caused difficulty that was often resolved by confining their interest to the first few results (we might identify this within critical literacy). Some adolescents in my team's study also noted the difficulty in retrieving relevant information,[32] but others felt that the Internet offered advantages over other sources, because some sites could personalize information (we might identify this within interactive literacy). Skinner et al[34] found that adolescents who use the Internet for health information felt that high-quality information did exist but that they were insufficiently skilled to find it (we might surmise that all aspects of health literacy contributed to this feeling).

Positive aspects of computer use, pointing toward possibilities for health-literacy improvement, are also present in recent studies. Valaitis[35] found that her sample of inner-city youth felt more empowered to communicate with adult care providers through this medium than through off-line channels, which is a facet of functional and interactive literacies. Nettleton et al[36] found that an interesting "concordance" is emerging between health information providers and consumers regarding the quality of online health information, which highlights critical literacy improvements; this has been a great concern among health professionals and policy makers, and perhaps their fears were unfounded as Internet use comes of age. Ybarra and Suman[37] explored behavior after accessing online health information in a national US survey including adolescents aged 12 years and older. They found that those who did not understand the information, perhaps through functional health literacy difficulties, sought peers to help them. This reminds us that the Internet is an additional source, and that the input of other informants is not supplanted; formal or informal "navigators" for adolescents, perhaps peers within school or trusted adults in the health care system, could still improve their health literacy skills.

The Internet, despite technologic breakthroughs in graphics and audiovisual interfaces, remains largely text driven. Adolescents, more than ever before, must acquire and develop literacy skills that allow them to be active information seekers. Not only do they have to read and comprehend the text before them, but they also have to construct their own key-word searches and e-mail messages to operate the most basic functions of the Web.

TO FILTER OR NOT TO FILTER?

At this point, it is worth reflecting on the issue of software filtering systems that are installed by parents and in many public-access places (schools, libraries, etc) to prevent exposure to sexually explicit material on the Web. Discussion about the use of filtering software in the United States has centered on how this method might not be perfect in blocking all inappropriate material.[38] It is also possible that it could actually block adolescents from getting information they need, for example, about sexual health and illicit drugs. A survey of Nebraska school board presidents revealed that they did not appreciate the negative impact that school Internet policies could have on access to health-education sites.[39] US commentators seem to be concluding that promoting parental and teacher involvement and discussion while young people search the Internet, so that adolescents develop their own discipline, may be a better solution than installing software.[40,41] The understandable tension between protecting adolescents and giving them access to health-education information is a major issue.

OPPORTUNITIES FOR IMPROVING ADOLESCENT HEALTH LITERACY USING THE INTERNET

Commentators have rightly concerned themselves with the "digital divide" regarding access to the Internet, but another, more insidious divide stems from adolescents' varying ability to effectively search for, evaluate, and apply the information they need to address a personal health concern. The demographic findings from the adults in the 2003 US NAAL could be useful indicators for reasons why some adolescents might have poor health literacy skills[14] and could be used to target adolescents to benefit from the REALM-Teen tool accompanied by some strategies to improve their skills.

HOW COULD THE INTERNET HELP ADOLESCENTS TO IMPROVE THEIR HEALTH LITERACY?

Recognizing that adolescents are interested in searching for online health information and that the Internet places demands on users that will test their health-literacy skills, it seems reasonable to propose that online tools for "diagnosis" and "treatment" of health-literacy deficits could help adolescents. In preparing this article, online adolescent-oriented tools to improve health literacy were sought, but none were found. Box 4 describes some off-line resources that might usefully be adapted for this purpose.

Practitioners should not underestimate the power of their own institution's Web sites as a place where teen-friendly tools, or links to such tools, could be placed. Those who have a teen clinic would be seen as a trusted source[26] by teens who are developing their critical online health literacy. All health care providers should assume that adolescents will search for health information online before, or after, a consultation. A working knowledge of some useful teen-friendly sites could enable providers to help adolescents to navigate more successfully and develop their skills (see Box 5 for some examples).

Box 4. Examples of off-line health literacy resources

- The Institute for Health Care Advancement Health Education Literacy Program (HELP) (www.hsph.harvard.edu/healthliteracy/curricula/for_health.html): the curriculum is aimed at adult parents and caregivers, but it includes a book (*What to Do for Teen Health*) that might usefully form the basis of a teen-friendly resource
- The University of Washington's "Teen Health and the Media" (http://depts.washington.edu/thmedia/view.cgi?section=aboutus): this is a media literacy intervention that includes health issues such as alcohol, smoking, and nutrition; drawing on Norman and Skinner's e-health literacy model,[24] this could form a useful junction between health, media, and online literacies
- DISCERN online tool (www.discern.org.uk): this information-evaluation tool could help consumers improve their critical literacy by providing criteria for judging the quality of the health information on a Web site[42]

CONCLUSIONS

The Internet has the potential to not only facilitate access to health information for adolescents but also help them develop health literacy skills that could be used both online and off-line. The popularity of the medium for teens, and its familiarity as a general information source, is no longer in doubt. Adolescents, however, must have fairly sophisticated literacy skills to access, evaluate, and use the large volume of information that is generated by a health-related search. The

---

Box 5. Examples of teen health Web sites

- KidsHealth teen pages (United States): www.kidshealth.org/teen
- Medline Plus (teen health) (United States): www.nlm.nih.gov/medlineplus/teenhealth.html
- Teen Health FX (United States): www.teenhealthfx.com
- FDA health information for Teens (United States): www.fda.gov/oc/opacom/kids/html/7teens.htm
- I wanna know (sexual health and sexuality) (United States): www.iwannaknow.org
- AskZen (United States: provider site in the Denver, CO, example): www.askzen.org
- Teenage Health Freak (United Kingdom): www.teenagehealthfreak.org
- Youth Health Talk (United Kingdom): www.youthhealthtalk.org

concept of e-health literacy is helpful,[24] because it proposes that an individual needs to have moderate skills across a range of literacies to maximize his or her benefit from this information source.

It has been noted that most current health literacy research and resources are not aimed at adolescents but, rather, at adults. One study by my team explored health literacy skills as they manifest themselves in adolescent Internet use, making explicit what other studies have implied.[32] Policy and practice have been stimulated by recent publications; more research is needed with adolescents to ensure that evidence-based health literacy interventions are available to them. Focusing health literacy research on an adolescent population allows health and education researchers, and curriculum developers, to use the formal education system to enhance generic literacy skills and use them as a foundation for discussing the specialist discourse and demands relating to health.

Young people already use this medium; thus, it would be feasible to have diagnostic online tools for self-testing of health literacy with subsequent therapeutic exercises to improve their skills. The teens in my team's study[32] had ideas for improving health Web sites aimed at their peers; user involvement from this Internet-savvy group would enhance interventions aimed at adolescents. It is vital that the advantages of the Internet as a medium be incorporated into such tools (large text, audio streaming, personalization) for teens with low general literacy to fully participate.

Although we anticipate and hope that an increase in health literacy skills will promote informed choice and subsequent adoption of health-promoting behaviors such as regular exercise, smoking cessation, and adherence to medications, we must accept that this will not always be the case. It is possible that, with access to a diverse range of online and off-line health information sources, a sophisticated user with high health literacy may conclude that the course of action best for them does not concur with the wishes of their providers or parents. As our understanding of health literacy matures, we must accept that there will be conflict. Health literacy extends beyond a simplistic practice model; trusting and accepting relationships between providers, parents, and adolescents will continue to be crucial to the health of young people.

It is essential that our efforts to understand and promote health literacy include teens. Their move toward independent decision-making and their development of health behaviors that will be maintained through adulthood could be positively influenced to reduce future poor health outcomes and the resultant pressure on health services. The Internet offers a convenient gateway to information that adolescents already use: we must seek to further understand the health literacy challenges that adolescents face and develop interventions that will be effective and relevant.

ACKNOWLEDGMENTS

My colleagues Jonathan Klein and Tracy Sesselberg (University of Rochester, Rochester, NY) and Peter Noyce and Judy Cantrill (University of Manchester, Manchester, England) were my partners in the adolescent Internet/health literacy studies. I thank them and the schools and students who took part. I thank Doris Gillis, CIHR Fellow and associate professor in the Department of Human Nutrition at St Francis Xavier University (Antigonish, Nova Scotia, Canada) for her most helpful comments during the drafting of this article. My adolescent Internet health information study was supported by the Commonwealth Fund, a private New York City–based foundation.

The views presented here are those of the author and not necessarily those of the Commonwealth Fund, its directors, officers, or staff.

REFERENCES

1. Moore DW, Bean TW, Birdyshaw D, Rycik JA. Adolescent literacy: a position statement. *J Adolesc Adult Lit.* 1999;43:97–112
2. Gray NJ, Klein JD. Adolescents and the Internet: health and sexuality information. *Curr Opin Obstet Gynecol.* 2006;18:519–524
3. Nielsen-Bohlman L, Panzer AM, Kindig DA, eds. *Health Literacy: A Prescription to End Confusion.* Washington DC: National Academies Press; 2004
4. US Department of Health and Human Services. *Healthy People 2010.* 2nd ed. With Understanding and Improving Health and Objectives for Improving Health. Washington, DC: US Government Printing Office; 2000
5. Ratzan SC, Parker RM. Introduction. In: Selden CR, Zorn M, Ratzan SC, Parker RM, eds. *National Library of Medicine Current Bibliographies in Medicine: Health Literacy.* Bethesda, MD: National Institutes of Health, US Department of Health and Human Services; 2000. NLM publication CBM 2000-1
6. World Health Organization. *Health Promotion Glossary.* Geneva, Switzerland: World Health Organization; 1998
7. Nutbeam D. Health literacy as a public health goal: a challenge for contemporary health education and communication strategies into the 21st century. *Health Promot Int.* 2000;15:259–267
8. Andrus MR, Roth MT. Health literacy: a review. *Pharmacotherapy.* 2002;22:282–302
9. Rudd RE, Moeykens BA, Colton TC. Health and literacy: a review of medical and public health literature. In: Cornings J, Garner B, Smith C, eds. *The Annual Review of Adult Learning and Literacy.* Vol 1. New York, NY: Jossey-Bass; 1999. Available at: http://ncsall.gse.harvard.edu/ann_rev/vol1_5.html. Accessed September 16, 2003
10. Davis TC, Crouch MA, Long SW, et al. Rapid assessment of literacy levels of adult primary care patients. *Fam Med.* 1991;23:433–435
11. Ad Hoc Committee on Health Literacy for the Council on Scientific Affairs, American Medical Association. Health literacy: report of the Council on Scientific Affairs. *JAMA.* 1999;281:552–557
12. Public Health Agency of Canada. What determines health? Available at: www.phac-aspc.gc.ca/ph-sp/phdd/determinants. Accessed December 15, 2006
13. Rootman I, Ronson B. Literacy and health research in Canada: where have we been and where should we go? *Can J Public Health.* 2005;96(suppl 2):S62–S77. Available at: www.nlhp.cpha.ca/lithlthe/lithlth.pdf. Accessed December 15, 2006

14. National Center for Education Statistics. *The Health Literacy of America's Adults: Results From the 2003 National Assessment of Adult Literacy.* Washington DC: National Center for Education Statistics; 2006. Available at: http://nces.ed.gov/pubs2006/2006483_1.pdf. Accessed December 7, 2006

15. Williams MV, Parker RM, Baker DW, Parikh NS, Pitkin K, Coates WC, Nurss JR. Inadequate functional health literacy among patients at two public hospitals. *JAMA.* 1995;274:1677–1682

16. Gazmararian JA, Parker RM, Baker DW. Reading skills and family planning knowledge and practices in a low-income managed-care population. *Obstet Gynecol.* 1999;93:239–244

17. Kalichman SC, Ramachandran B, Catz S. Adherence to combination antiretroviral therapies in HIV patients of low literacy. *J Gen Intern Med.* 1999;14:267–273

18. Baker DW, Parker RM, Williams MV, Clark S, Nurss J. The relationship of patient reading to self-reported health and use of health services. *Am J Public Health.* 1997;87:1027–1030

19. Schillinger D, Grumbach K, Piette J, et al. Association of health literacy with diabetes outcomes. *JAMA.* 2002;288:475–482

20. Weiss BD, Blanchard JS, McGee DL, et al. Illiteracy among Medicaid recipients and its relationship to health care costs. *J Health Care Poor Underserved.* 1994;5:99–111

21. Fortenberry JD, McFarlane MM, Hennessy M, et al. Relation of health literacy to gonorrhoea related care. *Sex Transm Infect.* 2001;77:206–211

22. Davis TC, Wolf MS, Arnold CL, et al. Development and validation of the Rapid Estimate of Adolescent Literacy in Medicine (REALM-Teen): a tool to screen adolescents for below-grade reading in health care settings. *Pediatrics.* 2006;118(6). Available at: www.pediatrics.org/cgi/content/full/118/6/e1707

23. University of Victoria Centre for Community Health Promotion Research. BC Literacy & Health Research Network: measurement of health literacy in schools. Available at: http://web.uvic.ca/chpc/whatwedo/research/lithealth/schoolliteracy.htm. Accessed December 14, 2006

24. Norman CD, Skinner HA. eHealth literacy: essential skills for consumer health in a networked world. *J Med Internet Res.* 2006;8:e9. Available at: www.jmir.org/2006/2/e9

25. Ackard DM, Neumark-Sztainer D. Health care information sources for adolescents: age and gender differences on use, concerns, and needs. *J Adolesc Health.* 2001;29:170–176

26. Gray NJ, Klein JD, Noyce PR, Sesselberg TS, Cantrill JA. Health information-seeking behaviour in adolescence: the place of the Internet. *Soc Sci Med.* 2005;60:1467–1478

27. Fox S. Pew Internet & American Life Project: online health search 2006. Available at: www.pewinternet.org/pdfs/PIP_Online_Health_2006.pdf. Accessed December 15, 2006

28. Borzekowski DLG, Rickert VI. Adolescent cybersurfing for health information: a new resource that crosses barriers. *Arch Pediatr Adolesc Med.* 2001;155:813–817

29. Rideout V. *Generation Rx.com: How Young People use the Internet for Health Information.* Menlo Park, CA: Kaiser Family Foundation; 2001

30. Goold PC, Ward M, Carlin EM. Can the Internet be used to improve sexual health awareness in Web-wise young people? *J Fam Plann Reprod Health Care.* 2003;29:28–30

31. Hanauer D, Dibble E, Fortin J, Col NF. Internet use among community college students: implications in designing healthcare interventions. *J Am Coll Health.* 2004;52:197–202

32. Gray NJ, Klein JD, Noyce PR, Sesselberg TS, Cantrill JA. The Internet: a window on adolescent health literacy. *J Adolesc Health.* 2005;37:243

33. Hansen DL, Derry HA, Resnick PJ, Richardson CR. Adolescents searching for health information on the Internet: an observational study. *J Med Internet Res.* 2003;5:e25. Available at: www.jmir.org/2003/4/e25

34. Skinner H, Biscope S, Poland B, Goldberg E. How adolescents use technology for health information: implications for health professionals from focus group studies. *J Med Internet Res.* 2003;5:e32. Available at: www.jmir.org/2003/4/e32

35. Valaitis RK. Computers and the Internet: tools for youth empowerment. *J Med Internet Res.* 2005;7:e51. Available at: www.jmir.org/2005/5/e51

36. Nettleton S, Burrows R, O'Malley L. The mundane realities of the everyday lay use of the Internet for health, and their consequences for media convergence. *Sociol Health Illn.* 2005;27:972–992

37. Ybarra ML, Suman M. Help seeking behavior and the Internet: a national survey. *Int J Med Inform.* 2006;75:29–41
38. Lenhart A. Pew Internet & American Life Project: protecting teens online. Available at www. pewinternet.org/pdfs/PIP_Filters_Report.pdf. Accessed December 15, 2006
39. Dennison D, Corbin D, Sharma M, Grandgenett N. Internet use policies and implications for health education: a survey of Nebraska School Board presidents. *Int Electron J Health Educ.* 2001;4:354–360
40. Iannotta JG, ed. *Nontechnical Strategies to Reduce Children's Exposure to Inappropriate Material on the Internet.* Washington, DC: National Academy Press; 2001
41. Gray NJ, Klein JD, Cantrill JA, Noyce PR. Adolescent girls' use of the Internet for health information: issues beyond access. *J Med Syst.* 2002;26:545–553
42. Charnock D, Shepperd S, Needham G, Gann R. DISCERN: an instrument for judging the quality of written consumer health information on treatment choices. *J Epidemiol Community Health.* 1999;53:105–111

Adolesc Med 18 (2007) 383–399

Using Interactive Behavior Change Technology to Intervene on Physical Activity and Nutrition With Adolescents

Leanne M. Mauriello, PhD*, Karen J. Sherman, BA,
Mary-Margaret H. Driskell, MPH,
Janice M. Prochaska, PhD

Pro-Change Behavior Systems, Inc, PO Box 755, West Kingston, RI 02892, USA

Interactive technologies have emerged as a promising means for developing and disseminating health behavior change interventions. Interactive health behavior change programs are most often computer-delivered via the World Wide Web, a CD-ROM/DVD, or a stand-alone kiosk. There are many benefits of programs using these technologies. They allow the incorporation of rich media such as audio, animated graphics, and video. On-screen assessments and programming allow for immediate feedback with extensive opportunities for tailoring to participant responses. The embedded interactivity gives the user an active role with more control over their participation. Users enjoy the appeal these features offer and the flexibility of engaging in the program at their convenience. Researchers and program implementers appreciate the fidelity to treatment offered with consistent and reliable feedback delivered to participants.[1] With improved program retention, wider reach, and less reliance on staff for delivery, interactive technologies offer a cost-effective means of delivering behavior change interventions.[2] They are acclaimed by researchers to be an innovative, powerful, and promising way of improving the efficacy and dissemination of behavior change interventions.[1,3–5]

Interactive technologies are particularly appealing for promoting health behaviors among youth.[6] Young populations welcome, almost demand, technology and multimedia products as constants in all arenas of their lives. They are accustomed to interactive learning and gaining knowledge through technology platforms. Hence, computer-delivered health promotion interventions need to be embraced as a means of reaching youth. The promotion of energy-balance behaviors among youth is one of the most timely and urgent public health priorities.[7,8] The grave

---

*Corresponding author.
E-mail address: lmauriello@prochange.com (L. M. Mauriello).

health consequences[9–13] and health care costs[14,15] associated with the growing epidemic of obesity have driven obesity prevention efforts, including promotion of physical activity and healthy dietary behaviors, to the forefront of youth health education and behavior change efforts. Interactive technologies are emerging as a way to complement, and even substitute for, the heavy reliance on curriculum-based interventions for physical activity and nutrition.[16–18] *Health in Motion*: *Healthy Teens, Healthy for Life*, detailed in "Case Study," is one example.[19]

BACKGROUND

Despite the need for promotion of health behaviors among adolescents[20,21] and their enthusiasm for interactive technologies,[18] surprisingly few computer-delivered behavior change interventions have been developed, particularly for high school students. The 11 published studies we reviewed[16,22–35] reveal many gaps and areas for expanding the use of interactive technologies for promoting physical activity and nutrition among adolescents. Of the 6 school-based interventions,[16,27–31,33,34] none were developed for high school students. Overall, school has been the delivery channel tested most often; only 1 intervention was tested in a primary care setting,[22–24] 1 was tested in a community-based organization,[32] and 3 were tested as primarily home-based programs.[25,26,35] The majority of the studies were not population based, but they instead targeted an at-risk group or a specific gender. In addition, the majority of the interventions were not tested as stand-alone programs but instead were tested in conjunction with direct contact.

Though many of the interventions were guided by a theoretical framework, few offered tailoring on theoretical constructs. Four of the interventions reviewed showed no behavioral changes,[25,31,33,35] and 2 others reflected a trend toward some behavioral impact through small-scale feasibility studies.[16,27] Among the 5 other studies, only modest outcomes have been reported, some being gender specific, short-term, or within sedentary behavior instead of physical activity.[24,26,30,32,34]

One of the studies we reviewed requires a slightly closer examination because of its relevance to current research. The Patient-Centered Assessment and Counseling for Exercise + Nutrition (PACE+) program is an interactive computer program that targets physical activity, dietary fat, fruit and vegetable consumption, and sedentary behavior for adolescents in a primary care setting.[22–24] Adolescent participants receive tailored feedback and action plans to share with their providers. In a randomized, controlled trial of 878 adolescents aged 11 to 15 years, PACE+, when coupled with 12 months of telephone counseling and mailings, significantly reduced sedentary behaviors among boys and girls compared with those in the control group.[24] In addition, there was improvement in the proportion of adolescents meeting recommended health guidelines compared with those in the control group. PACE+ did not demonstrate between-group differences for other behavioral indicators or for BMI.

Despite the modest outcomes, PACE+ is an important example of using interactive technology with adolescents. As the first randomized, controlled trial of a program applying interactive technology in these behavioral areas, it is quite notable that the PACE+ intervention demonstrated significant effects across multiple behaviors, was feasible to implement in primary care settings, and was shown to be acceptable among teens.[22] PACE+ is the most promising adolescent physical activity/nutrition intervention for dissemination in a primary care setting. It serves as a model for future program development.

With work in this area only in its infancy, our review of published literature points to the many areas left for additional investigation and development. The following case example of a multimedia obesity prevention program currently in trial highlights the development of a high school–based program.

CASE STUDY: *HEALTH IN MOTION*

Health in Motion is a computer-delivered multimedia obesity prevention program for high school students that promotes physical activity (≥ 60 minutes of physical activity ≥ 5 days/week), fruit and vegetable consumption (≥ 5 servings of fruits and vegetables per day), and limited television viewing (≤ 2 hours/ day).[19] Although the long-term goal of *Health in Motion* is obesity prevention, its main objective is to help all students, regardless of weight, adopt and maintain these 3 healthy behaviors. Students interact with the program through a series of transtheoretical model (TTM)–based assessments and tailored feedback messages. Multimedia components, including audio, video, and Flash animations, help to capture the students' interest.

The TTM integrates 4 theoretical constructs: stage of change, decisional balance (pros and cons), self-efficacy (confidence), and processes of change (behavioral and experiential processes).[36–38] The TTM is used as an overarching framework to determine the stage-appropriate constructs for which to deliver feedback. For *Health in Motion* to be completed within 1 class period, and so that it does not overwhelm participants, a full TTM intervention is delivered for physical activity, in which each of the constructs of the TTM is addressed. Optimally, tailored interventions are given for fruit and vegetable consumption and limited television viewing. Tailored interventions offer limited feedback representing the most-important TTM constructs for the respective stage of change for a specific behavior. In addition to the interactive student intervention, staff and family guides were developed to inform teachers, administrators, and family members about the intervention, target behaviors, and strategies for helping teens with behavior change. Table 1 summarizes 10 key features of *Health in Motion*.

Table 1
Key features of *Health in Motion*

Feature	Description
Population based	Relevant for all high school students regardless of weight or readiness to change target behaviors
Addresses multiple behaviors	Promotes physical activity, consumption of fruits and vegetables, and limited television viewing according to national guidelines
Theory based	TTM is used as overarching framework for decision rules and all program content
Tailored content	Expert-system technology offers participants standardized and individualized normative and ipsative feedback based on their responses to salient variables
Computer delivered	Accessible via the Internet; can be loaded onto a DVD or personal computer
Uses interactive technology	Participants control the pace of the program and have opportunities to type in responses and select strategies they want to use
Multimedia	Incorporates audio, video, Flash animations, and captivating images
Designed from formative research	Focus groups with students, individual interviews with students and experts, expert reviews, and a student pilot test helped shape the final program
Designed for easy dissemination	Self-directed, stand-alone computer program fits within a 30-min class period; requires little to no staff training and allows for low-cost and consistent delivery across dissemination channels
Flexible dissemination	Can be disseminated in classroom settings (such as health or physical education), as part of a wellness program, at youth or community organizations, in health care settings, by health care insurers, or by school nurses or primary care providers

Use of Technology

Health in Motion is an expert system intervention. Expert systems are broadly defined as computer programs that mimic the reasoning and problem solving of human "experts."[39] Expert systems are programmed to provide expert advice using statistical decision-making rules. The decision-making rules for *Health in Motion* were determined from statistical analyses conducted on a large, normative, measurement development database gathered during formative research and theoretical algorithms based on the TTM. *Health in Motion* is currently accessible via the Internet (www.prochange.com/obesitydemo). The program also can be loaded on a DVD or personal computer.

The expert system intervention relies on the integration of statistical, multimedia, and database software to provide users with individualized, tailored feedback. The proprietary software is a Java application that accesses the rules defined in the program files to give TTM-based, individualized feedback. Once a participant starts answering assessment questions, immediate, on-screen tailored feedback is provided based on the user's responses, stage of change, and preprogrammed algorithms. These feedback files appear in the form of text, graphics, Flash animations, and videos.

In a baseline intervention session, the expert system compares a participant's responses to a large, comparative sample of other individuals in the same stage of change (normative comparisons) and provides individualized feedback to facilitate forward stage movement. All subsequent follow-up sessions are based on comparisons to both the normative group (comparisons to others) and the individual's own previous responses (ipsative or self-comparison). Ipsative feedback, which involves access to a database of results of previous contacts with that individual, reinforces progress that individuals have made since their last assessment and outlines specific steps they can take to progress further or prevent relapse.[40]

The expert system offers highly individualized feedback to each participant.[41] *Health in Motion* offers >300 unique feedback combinations at baseline and >33 000 unique sessions at follow-up. The expert system serves as a surrogate counselor using statistical decision-making to guide the participant through the intricacies of each stage, encouraging the use of the most appropriate processes of change. This enables a level of standardization and fidelity to the treatment that is not possible with curriculum-based, lecture-based, or counseling-based interventions.[42] This population-based intervention modality also enables a much wider reach in a cost-effective manner.

Interactive and multimedia components are critical for making the expert system intervention engaging to adolescents and relaying important information about the target behaviors. The welcome screen begins with an image slide show depicting teens performing the target behaviors while upbeat music is played. The image slide show ends with a static image of ordinary teens depicting the target behaviors (Fig 1). Throughout the program, unique depictions of teens and the target behaviors are used as much as possible, with image slide shows scattered throughout the program. A diverse set of teens narrate the program and read all on-screen text. At each session, 2 or 3 stage-matched videos (45 seconds to 2 minutes in length) show teens discussing the target behaviors and modeling important behavior change strategies such as helping relationships, stimulus control, and consciousness raising. Throughout the program, Flash movies and animations are incorporated as introductions to new sections or as part of feedback messages. For example, one screen shows the benefits of eating fruits and vegetables flying onto the screen as teens read them.

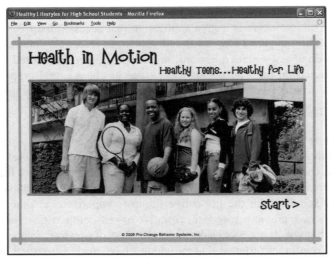

Fig 1. Screen shot of teens depicting target behaviors.

Health in Motion is an interactive program, because users are active participants. Users interact with the program by answering assessment questions about their attitudes and behaviors. On assessment screens, users control the narration by enabling audio as desired. Users can also relay their own ideas in on-screen type-in fields or click in boxes to "check off" the presented strategies that they plan to use. Finally, users are in control of their progress through the program because they choose when to move from screen to screen.

User Experience

After the welcome screen loads, users are asked to log in to the program and provide assent. Depending on whether they are completing a baseline or follow-up session, users begin the program by viewing either a Flash movie that shows teens with quotes about the target behaviors or a video introduction that welcomes them back. Next, the teen narrators introduce the program and try to capture the user's attention by introducing what will be covered and relating it to teens. The program then proceeds through the physical activity, fruit and vegetable, and television viewing sections, alternating between assessments and tailored feedback messages. Each behavioral section ends with a summary of stage-specific strategies. The program concludes with an overall summary, which includes integrated feedback on stages of change across the 3 behaviors and stage-based next steps for each behavior. A demonstration of the program can be viewed at www.prochange.com/obesitydemo.

Although much of the intervention content appears on-screen as text, the activities and strategies vary to keep the user's attention and to relate the information

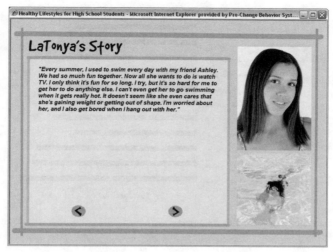

Fig 2. Screen shot of a testimonial.

in meaningful and persuasive ways. There are brief, animated introductions to break up each behavioral section. Within a section, factual information is presented in the form of debunking myths, giving fun facts, and miniquizzes. Quotes from teens are interspersed throughout the program. In addition, to meet the recommendations of teens, concrete examples are given for ways to eat fruits and vegetables when eating out, ways to be active while watching television, and ideas for getting enough physical activity in poor weather conditions or in urban environments. Testimonies are offered throughout the program in which students hear about another teen's experience in overcoming a barrier with one of the target behaviors (Fig 2). Finally, all feedback paragraphs were written to be appropriate for the cognitive ability, reading level, and general perspectives of adolescents. For instance, strategies for adding more physical activity to their day include suggestions such as walking home from school or to a friend's house, participating in extracurricular activities, and getting their family involved in more activity.

Acceptability Outcomes/Effectiveness Trial

As part of a Phase I Small Business Innovation Research grant, a pilot test was conducted in May 2004 with 45 students (11th and 12th grades) at a New England high school. Pilot-test participants rated the program very positively (see ref 19 for full review of pilot results). On a 5-point scale (1 = strongly disagree; 5 = strongly agree), students gave the program an average score of ≥3.60 on all 12 dimensions. Figure 3 shows the percentage of students who responded that they strongly agree or agree with each evaluation dimension. The usability of the program was its strongest feature, with an overwhelming majority of participants

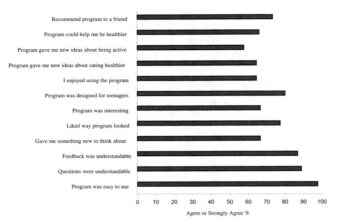

Fig 3. Acceptability results from the pilot test.

strongly agreeing or agreeing that the program was easy to use, and that the questions and feedback were easy to understand. The content, look and feel, and age-appropriateness also were highly rated by participants. Nearly 75% of participants responded that they would recommend the program to a friend. Pilot-test participants also offered qualitative feedback to 4 open-ended questions. Understanding what they liked most and least about the program, why they would or would not recommend it to a friend, and what they would change about the program offered insight into how the Phase II product should be changed and enhanced.

During development of *Health in Motion*, a variety of experts and school personnel (including specialists in cultural diversity, pediatric wellness and primary care, health and physical education, and school administration) reviewed the program. These experts found the program engaging, acceptable, and "much needed" in high schools.

The successful implementation and completion of the intervention within a 30-minute class period during the pilot test confirmed the feasibility and suitability of *Health in Motion* for the school setting. As part of a Phase II Small Business Innovation Research grant, an effectiveness trial of *Health in Motion* is currently underway in 8 schools nationwide. Schools in the trial are assigned to either (1) the intervention group that receives the complete *Health in Motion* intervention once per month for 3 months or (2) the control group that receives assessments only. Both groups will complete follow-up assessments at 6 months and 1 year postintervention to compare changes in physical activity, fruit and vegetable consumption, television viewing, and BMI. Students and school personnel involved in the treatment group also will be asked to complete an evaluation measure to assess the acceptability of the Phase II program.

CONCLUSIONS AND FUTURE DIRECTIONS

The review of existing interactive physical activity and nutrition interventions for adolescents and lessons learned through the development of *Health in Motion* offer insight for future intervention designs. The most obvious result of the literature review is that much more research and program development should be devoted to this area. Innovation is sorely needed to address the lack of adequate physical activity and nutrition among adolescents and to prevent the decline of these behaviors into adulthood.[43,44] A large, measurement development survey conducted for Phase I of *Health in Motion* validates this priority. Among the 1459 high school students surveyed, 63% were in a preaction stage (not currently performing the behavior) for doing ≥60 minutes of physical activity ≥5 days/week; 89% were in a preaction stage for eating ≥5 servings of fruits and vegetables per day; and 46.7% were in a preaction stage for limiting television viewing to ≤2 hours/day. Looking across behaviors, only 4.7% were at risk (in a preaction stage) for 0 behaviors and 22.5% for 1 behavior, whereas 42.1% were at risk for 2 and 30.6% were at risk for all 3 behaviors.[45] Clearly, increasing physical activity and healthy dietary practices should be a focal point for adolescent health promotion efforts. But where should research be directed, and what lessons can be shared to guide the field toward the development of appropriate, acceptable, and efficacious interventions? Five overarching areas to guide future development will be discussed: (1) the need to reach and intervene with older adolescents; (2) incorporating formative research in development; (3) using flexible and cost-effective delivery platforms; (4) overcoming obstacles faced with testing and disseminating interactive programs in schools; and (5) aiming for the highest impact by offering a theory-grounded, tailored, and population-based approach.

From the published literature, we see that high school students have been understudied as a target population for the development of interactive health behavior change interventions. Schools present an optimal way through which to reach large numbers of culturally and socioeconomically diverse students.[46,47] High schools need to be additionally used as a way to promote physical activity and nutrition among adolescents before the start of adulthood and the likely decline in these behavioral areas. Research conducted in this area confirms that high school students find interactive interventions acceptable and appealing.[19, 16,22] Thus, older adolescents should welcome teen-appropriate interactive interventions.

Toward this end, formative research can be used as a way to connect with the target audience and plan for the development of an intervention that will be relevant for, and appealing to, the audience. This is important when adult researchers are developing a program for teens, a population for which the latest social trends and cutting-edge technologies are important. One expert who reviewed *Health in Motion* proclaimed that, "the greatest thing is that I didn't think the kids would think it was hokey or stupid." The development of *Health in Motion* involved focus groups and cognitive interviews with students, individual interviews with school personnel and administrators, and expert reviews. The goal of these formative activities was to create a program acceptable to students and marketable to schools. Some of the most important lessons learned from students are presented in Table 2. In addition to involving students in the development of *Health in Motion*, we found that involving key informants and potential buyers in the design phase increased our chances of creating a product that is acceptable and able to be disseminated easily. Through this process, we learned of the need to balance the wishes of the students and the needs of the potential buyers with the development of a science-based intervention.

Although schools have been the delivery channel used most frequently in published studies thus far, the integration of interactive interventions in the school environment can present challenges. There are wide discrepancies in the technologic capabilities of schools. Whereas some schools have new hardware and efficient network connectivity, many schools struggle to stay up-to-date with technology. To accommodate this, the development of interactive interventions for delivery in schools needs to begin with an assessment of the technology available in schools. Design teams should include experts in computer programming, networking, and multimedia delivery. The system requirements of the intervention need to balance the desire for highly interactive and multimedia-intensive features with the reality of the schools' technologic capabilities.[48]

Furthermore, some schools struggle to have enough computers for >1 class of students to use simultaneously. This can pose challenges when physical activity and nutrition interventions are delivered during health or physical education classes, because these classes typically do not meet in classrooms with computers. This requires additional coordination and possible rearrangement of schedules to reserve computer laboratories. Researchers can overcome this barrier by providing laptop computers; however, this hinders the ability to test the intervention in real-world circumstances.

Tracking students across multiple years also can pose challenges for this research. Across schools, there is variation in the frequency and length of health and physical education courses, particularly when these classes are offered as electives. Within high school samples, researchers also face more transience, because students are more likely to transfer or drop out than younger students.[49] When conducting research, it can help to connect research staff to schools to assist with student tracking and retention. Researchers and schools can collaborate to overcome the obstacles faced with conducting school-based research on interactive interventions.

The review of existing interactive interventions to promote adolescent physical activity and nutrition reveals the need to expand the use of a variety of dissem-

Table 2

Key lessons learned from high school students for developing an acceptable intervention

Lessons Learned	Teens' Quotes
Use captivating images	
Use new images on each screen	"We want to see things in motion—the people should be doing things."
Use bright and engaging images	"The pictures should all be bright, bold, and colorful."
Depict realistic teens doing the behaviors	"Show us ideas of things we could do other than watching TV."
Display options for how to perform the target behaviors	
Develop a program for teens, by teens	
Let participants know that you interviewed teens when developing the program	"Say something about interviewing teens—that you got actual information from teens not just a bunch of information adults put together as usual. Let them know you heard what goes on in our lives."
Use quotes from teens throughout the program	
Give specific strategies	
Give concrete suggestions for performing the target behaviors	"Give 'how to' guidance when it comes to doing the target behaviors."
Offer tips and take-home messages	"Overall I think it was good; the facts and tips were the most important parts."
Make it entertaining	
Do things to capture their attention	"Have something to catch our attention—did they really say that?"
Provide shocking statistics	"If we see famous people do it, we'll want to, too."
Use animations	"We want to see videos and music—spark our interest right away."
Make it interactive	
Have type-in boxes and opportunities to check things off	"If I can't click on it, I don't like it." "Have things we can fill in, so we can plan out how we're going to do [the target behaviors]."
Make the tailoring obvious	
Be explicit that the messages are personalized for teens	"There has to be something good in it for us, otherwise kids will think there's too much work in it." "I like that the program tells you new things and where you were before and now. Say that somewhere."
Focus on behaviors, not disease prevention	
Students are interested, to some extent, in improving their health behavior, but they do not feel susceptible to disease	"Obesity is too outrageous—we're not even close to being obese. Getting chunky is what we're worried about."

ination channels. Interventions with flexible dissemination possibilities will in-crease opportunities for dissemination and enable testing of various delivery channels. Pace+ was created for the primary care setting; however, Prochaska et al[34] also used a modified version of Pace+ in the school environment. Although *Health in Motion* is being tested in schools, the Web-based platform allows for many dissemination possibilities. *Health in Motion* could be accessed as a kiosk in a primary care setting, or it could be accessed via personal computers in a home or community setting, such as the Boys & Girls Clubs. Flexible dissemi-nation allows for the widest possible reach and the greatest possible impact.

Aiming for wide reach and high impact, interventions are needed with a popu-lation-based approach, similar to that of *Health in Motion*. Although designing an intervention that targets a specific gender, culture, or at-risk group can serve an important purpose, population-based approaches that can be disseminated widely are particularly needed for the promotion of physical activity and nutrition.[18,50,51] Messages about these behaviors must reach all teens, regardless of weight or demographic characteristics. These behaviors are underpracticed by the majority of adolescents and are important determinants of future disease trends across the entire population.

Ease of dissemination is an important feature in the development of all interven-tions.[52] Interactive interventions have the ability to serve as stand-alone inter-vention components without the reliance on staff for delivery of curriculum-based intervention materials.[53] Given the potential for cost reduction and ease of dissemination, the utility and efficacy of interactive interventions as stand-alone components needs to be examined. The majority of research included in this literature review combined an interactive intervention with another intervention component, most often face-to-face interaction with staff. *Health in Motion* is one example of a Web-based physical activity and nutrition intervention being tested as a stand-alone program. More research is needed to compare the efficacy and cost-effectiveness of the delivery of adolescent programs that are solely Web based with those that are part of a multicomponent intervention. The cost-effectiveness of implementing interactive interventions in isolation will be an important aspect to consider.

An important feature of the development of effective interactive interventions is the ability to tailor participant feedback.[54,55] The majority of programs reviewed did incorporate some level of tailoring, although many did not offer tailoring based on theoretical constructs. A solid behavior change theory should serve as a framework to guide the development of an intervention.[56,57] Science-based interventions that use key principles of behavior change theory to tailor feedback can advance the field. The theoretically tailored interventions of Patrick et al[24] and Frenn et al[30] produced the most promising outcomes of the programs reviewed. Still, even these interventions offered individually tailored feedback only on stage of change. Similar to *Health in Motion*, interactive interventions should be used to offer individually tailored feedback on as many theoretical constructs as possible.[40,55,58]

Prochaska and colleagues[34] concern of intervening on multiple risks within adolescent populations is valid, but strategies can be used to overcome the possible burden of multiple-behavior interventions. Interestingly, some interventions reviewed found significant changes in sedentary behavior despite not addressing sedentary behavior specifically. Research has linked sedentary behavior to weight concerns.[59–61] Dietary practices are poorer among those with higher rates of television viewing,[62,63] and those who are sedentary are less likely to engage in an adequate amount of physical activity.[64,65] Sedentary behavior may be an important behavior to combine within physical activity and nutrition interventions, particularly when the focus is obesity prevention. Optimally, tailored interventions, such as *Health in Motion*, can offer the most important feedback on multiple behaviors while keeping the amount of feedback manageable. There is growing evidence for the efficacy of multiple behavior interventions.[66–68] Energy-balance behaviors are intrinsically related, and multiple behavior interventions will allow researchers to treat these behaviors as such while allowing for potentially greater impacts. Future research is needed to determine the most effective way to address multiple behaviors within interactive physical activity and nutrition programs for adolescents.

The most disappointing result of the published reviews of interactive adolescent interventions for physical activity and nutrition is the inconsistent and modest findings of the work done to date. Much of the intervention development thus far has included only small-scale feasibility studies and nonrandomized trials, and many have not included the important characteristic of tailoring based on theoretical constructs. Even the best of outcomes produced only modest findings.[24,26,30] However, as this area of intervention development expands and enhances, more impressive outcomes are likely to result. Research on the development of interactive interventions for physical activity and nutrition among adult and elementary school populations shows promise, as does the use of interactive technologies for health behavior change in other areas.[69–74] The success of TTM-based, computer-delivered multimedia bullying-prevention interventions that were designed and implemented similarly to *Health in Motion* offer great promise that the acceptability of *Health in Motion* will lead to efficacious outcomes. These middle school and high school bullying-prevention interventions showed significant treatment effects; bullying behavior was reduced by 30% among middle school students and 40% among high school students.[75] If proven effective, the development and delivery of *Health in Motion* can be an efficient, low-cost, population-based example of interactive technology to promote physical activity, fruit and vegetable consumption, and limited television viewing among adolescents.

ACKNOWLEDGMENT

This work was supported by grant R43 HL074482 from the National Heart, Lung, and Blood Institute.

REFERENCES

1. Fotheringham M, Owies D, Leslie E, Owen N. Interactive health communication in preventive medicine: internet-based strategies in teaching and research. *Am J Prev Med*. 2000;19:113–120
2. Wantland D, Portillo C, Holzemer W, Slaughter R, McGhee E. The effectiveness of Web-based vs. non-Web-based interventions: a meta-analysis of behavioral change outcomes. *J Med Internet Res*. 2004;6(4):e40. Available at: www.jmir.org/2004/4/e40
3. Marshall A, Owen N, Bauman A. Mediated approaches for influencing physical activity: update of the evidence on mass media, print, telephone, and website delivery of interventions. *J Sci Med Sport*. 2004;7:74–80
4. Atkinson N, Gold R. The promise and challenge of eHealth interventions. *Am J Health Behav*. 2002;26:494–503
5. Freimuth V, Quinn S. The contributions of health communication to eliminating health disparities. *Am J Public Health*. 2004;94:2053–2055
6. Gray N, Klein J, Noyce P, Sesselberg T, Cantrill J. Health information-seeking behavior in adolescence: the place of the internet. *Soc Sci Med*. 2005;60:1467–1478
7. US Department of Health and Human Services. *Surgeon General's Call to Action to Prevent and Decrease Overweight and Obesity*. Rockville, MD: US Department of Health and Human Services, Public Health Service, Office of the Surgeon General; 2001
8. US Department of Health and Human Services. Understanding mechanisms of health risk behavior change in children and adolescents. Available at: http://grants.nih.gov/grants/guide/pafiles/PA-04-121.html. Accessed July 6, 2004
9. US Department of Health and Human Services. Overweight and obesity: health consequences. Available at: www.surgeongeneral.gov/topics/obesity/calltoaction/fact_consequences.htm. Accessed July 3, 2007
10. Willett W, Manson J, Stampfer M, et al. Weight, weight change, and coronary heart disease in women: risk within the "normal" weight range. *JAMA*. 1995;273:461–465
11. Muntner P, He J, Cutler J, Wildman R, Whelton P. Trends in blood pressure among children and adolescents. *JAMA*. 2004;291:2107–2113
12. Gilliland F, Berhane K, Islam T, et al. Obesity and the risk of newly diagnosed asthma in school-age children. *Am J Epidemiol*. 2003;158:406–415
13. Must A, Strauss R. Risks and consequences of childhood and adolescent obesity. *Int J Obes Relat Metab Disord*. 1999;23(suppl 2):S2–S11
14. National Institute for Health Care Management. *Obesity in Young Children: Impact and Intervention*. Washington, DC: National Institute for Health Care Management Foundation; 2004
15. Finkelstein EA, Fiebelkorn IC, Wang G. National medical spending attributable to overweight and obesity: how much, and who's paying? *Health Aff (Millwood)*. 2003;(suppl):W3–219–226. Available at: http://content.healthaffairs.org/cgi/reprint/hlthaff.w3.219v1
16. Long J, Armstrong M, Amos E, et al. Pilot using World Wide Web to prevent diabetes in adolescents. *Clin Nurs Res*. 2006;15:67–79
17. Geiger B, Petri C, Myers O, et al. Using technology to teach health: a collaborative pilot project in Alabama. *J Sch Health*. 2002;72:401–407
18. Baranowski T, Cullen K, Nicklas T, Thompson D, Baranowski J. School-based obesity prevention: a blueprint for taming the epidemic. *Am J Health Behav*. 2002;26:486–493
19. Mauriello L, Driskell M, Sherman K, Johnson S, Prochaska JM, Prochaska JO. Acceptability of a school-based intervention for the prevention of adolescent obesity. *J Sch Nurs*. 2006;22:269–277

20. Dietz W, Gortmaker S. Preventing obesity in children and adolescents. *Annu Rev Public Health.* 2001;22:337–353

21. Mendlein J, Baranowski T, Pratt M. Physical activity and nutrition in children and youth: opportunities for performing assessments and conducting interventions. *Prev Med.* 2000;31: S150–S153

22. Prochaska J, Zabinski M, Calfas K, Sallis J, Patrick K. Pace+: interactive communication technology for behavior change in clinical settings. *Am J Prev Med.* 2000;19:127–131

23. Patrick K, Sallis J, Prochaska J, et al. A multicomponent program for nutrition and physical activity change in primary care. *Arch Pediatr Adolesc Med.* 2001;155:940–946

24. Patrick K, Calfas K, Norman G, et al. Randomized controlled trial of a primary care and home-based intervention for physical activity and nutrition behaviors. *Arch Pediatr Adolesc Med.* 2006;160:128–136

25. Abroms L, Fagan P, Eisenberg M, Lee H, Remva N, Sorensen G. The STRENGTH Ezine: an application of e-mail for health promotion in adolescent girls. *Am J Health Promot.* 2004;19: 28–32

26. Williamson D, Walden H, White M, et al. Two-year internet-based randomized controlled trial for weight loss in African-American girls. *Obesity (Silver Spring).* 2006;14:1231–1243

27. Horowitz M, Shilts M, Townsend M. EatFit: a goal-oriented intervention that challenges adolescents to improve their eating and fitness choices. *J Nutr Educ Behav.* 2004;36:43–44

28. Horowitz M, Shilts M, Townsend M. Adapting a diet analysis program for an adolescent audience. *J Nutr Educ Behav.* 2005;37:43–44

29. Frenn M, Malin S, Bansal N, et al. Addressing health disparities in middle school students' nutrition and exercise. *J Community Health Nurs.* 2003;20:1–14

30. Frenn M, Malin S, Brown R, et al. Changing the tide: an Internet/video exercise and low-fat diet intervention with middle-school students. *Appl Nurs Res.* 2005;18:13–21

31. Robbins L, Gretebeck K, Kazanis A, Pender N. Girls on the Move program to increase physical activity participation. *Nurs Res.* 2006;55:206–216

32. Jago R, Baranowski T, Baranowski J, et al. Fit for Life Boy Scout Badge: outcome evaluation of a troop and Internet intervention. *Prev Med.* 2006;42:181–187

33. Long J, Stevens K. Using technology to promote self-efficacy for healthy eating in adolescents. *J Nurs Scholarsh.* 2004;36:134–139

34. Prochaska J, Sallis J. A randomized controlled trial of single versus multiple health behavior change: promoting activity and nutrition among adolescents. *Health Psychol.* 2004;23:314–318

35. Marks J, Campbell M, Ward D, Ribisl K, Wildemuth B, Symons M. A comparison of Web and print media for physical activity promotion among adolescent girls. *J Adolesc Health.* 2006;39: 96–104

36. Prochaska J, DiClemente C. Stages and processes of self-change of smoking: toward an integrative model of change. *J Consult Clin Psychol.* 1983;51:390–395

37. Prochaska J, Velicer W, Rossi J, et al. Stages of change and decisional balance for 12 problem behaviors. *Health Psychol.* 1994;13:39–46

38. Prochaska J, Velicer W, DiClemente C, Fava J. Measuring processes of change: applications to the cessation of smoking. *J Consult Clin Psychol.* 1988;56:520–528

39. Negotia U. *Expert Systems and Fuzzy Systems.* Menlo Park, CA: Benjamin/Cummings; 1985

40. De Vries H, Brug J. Computer tailored interventions motivating people to adopt health promoting behaviors: introduction to a new approach. *Patient Educ Couns.* 1999;36:99–105

41. Marcus B, Nigg C, Riebe D, Forsyth L. Interactive communication strategies: implications for population-based physical-activity promotion. *Am J Prev Med.* 2000;19:121–126

42. Brug J, Oenema A, Campbell M. Past, present, and future of computer tailored nutrition education. *Am J Clin Nutr.* 2003;77(4 suppl):1028S–1034S

43. Munoz K, Krebs-Smith S, Ballard-Barbash R, Cleveland L. Food intake of US children and adolescents compared with recommendations. *Pediatrics.* 1997;100:323–329

44. Pate RR, Freedson RS, Sallis JF, et al. Compliance with physical activity guidelines: prevalence in a population of children and youth. *Ann Epidemiol.* 2002;12:303–308

45. Driskell M, Mauriello L, Sherman K. Using the transtheoretical model from childhood to adolescence: examining readiness for obesity prevention behaviors. Presented at: 134th Annual Meeting of the American Public Health Association; November 8, 2006; Boston, MA

46. Owen N, Glanz K, Sallis J, Kelder S. Evidence-based approaches to dissemination and diffusion of physical activity interventions. *Am J Prev Med.* 2006;31(4 suppl):S35–S44

47. Pyle S. Fighting an epidemic: the role of schools in reducing childhood obesity. *Psychol Sch.* 2006;43:361–376

48. Danaher B, Jazdzewski S, McKay H, Hudson C. Bandwith constraints to using video and other rich media in behavior change websites. *J Med Internet Res.* 2005;7:e49. Available at: www.jmir.org/2005/4/e49

49. Roderick M, Camburn E. Risk and recovery from course failure in the early years of high school. *Am Educ Res J.* 1999;36:303–343

50. Eng T. Population health technologies: emerging innovations for the health of the public. *Am J Prev Med.* 2004;26:237–242

51. Kohn M, Rees J, Brill S, et al. Preventing and treating adolescent obesity: a position paper of the Society for Adolescent Medicine. *J Adolesc Health.* 2006;38:784–787

52. Glasgow R, Vogt T, Boles S. Evaluating the public health impact of health promotion interventions: the RE-AIM framework. *Am J Public Health.* 1999;89:1322–1327

53. Marcus B, Owen N, Forsyth L, Cavill N, Fridinger F. Physical activity interventions using mass media, print media, and information technology. *Am J Prev Med.* 1998;15:362–378

54. Ruiter R, Kessels L, Jansma B, Brug J. Increased attention for computer-tailored health communications: an event-related potential study. *Health Psychol.* 2006;25:300–306

55. Kreuter M, Strecher V, Glassman B. One size does not fit all: the case for tailoring print materials. *Ann Behav Med.* 1999;21:276–283

56. Steckler A, Allegrante J, Altman D, et al. Health education intervention strategies: recommendations for future research. *Health Educ Q.* 1995;22:307–328

57. Prochaska JO, Prochaska JM. An update on maximum impact practices from a transtheoretical approach. In: Trafton JA, Gordon WP, eds. *Best Practices in the Behavioral Management of Chronic Diseases.* Vol 1. Los Altos, CA: Institute for Disease Management; 2003:1–16

58. Prochaska, J. Moving beyond the transtheoretical model. *Addictions.* 2006;101:768–774

59. Lowry R, Wechsler H, Galuska D, Fulton J, Kann L. Television viewing and its associations with overweight, sedentary lifestyle, and insufficient consumption of fruits and vegetables among US high school students. *J Sch Health.* 2002;72:413–421

60. Epstein L, Paluch R, Kilanowski C, Raynor H. The effect of reinforcement or stimulus control to reduce sedentary behavior in the treatment of pediatric obesity. *Health Psychol.* 2004;23:371–380

61. Hu F, Li T, Colditz G, Willett W, Manson J. Television watching and other sedentary behaviors in relation to risk of obesity and type 2 diabetes mellitus in women. *JAMA.* 2003;289:1785–1791

62. Robinson T, Killen J. Ethnic and gender differences in the relationships between television viewing and obesity, physical activity, and dietary fat intake. *J Health Educ.* 2005;26:S91–S98

63. Boynton-Jarret T, Ptereson K, Wiecha J, Sobol A, Gortmaker S. Impact of television viewing patterns on fruit and vegetable consumption among adolescents. *Pediatrics.* 2003;112:1321–1326

64. Koezuka N, Koo M, Allison K, et al. The relationship between sedentary activities and physical inactivity among adolescents: results from the Canadian Community Health Survey. *J Adolesc Health.* 2006;39:515–522

65. Santos M, Gomes H, Mota J. Physical activity and sedentary behaviors in adolescents. *Ann Behav Med.* 2005;30:21–24

66. Emmons K, McBride C, Puleo E, et al. Project PREVENT: a randomized trial to reduce multiple behavioral risk factors for colon cancer. *Cancer Epidemiol Biomarkers Prev.* 2005;14:1453–1459

67. Prochaska J, Velicer W, Redding C, et al. Stage-based expert systems to guide a population of primary care patients to quit smoking, eat healthier, prevent skin cancer, and receive regular mammograms. *Prev Med.* 2005;41:406–416

68. Johnson S, Driskell M, Johnson J, Prochaska JM, Zwick W, Prochaska JO. Efficacy of a transtheoretical model-based expert system for antihypertensive adherence. *Dis Manag.* 2006; 9:291–301
69. Baranowski T, Baranowski J, Cullen K, et al. Squire's Quest! Dietary outcome evaluation of a multimedia game. *Am J Prev Med.* 2003;24:52–61
70. Goran M, Reynolds K. Interactive multimedia for promoting physical activity (IMPACT) in children. *Obes Res.* 2005;13:762–771
71. Oenema A, Brug J, Lechner L. Web based tailored nutrition education: results of a randomized control trial. *Health Educ Res.* 2001;16:647–660
72. Napolitano M, Fotheringham M, Tate D, et al. Evaluation of an Internet based physical activity intervention: a preliminary investigation. *Ann Behav Med.* 2003;25:92–99
73. Tate D, Wing R, Winett R. Using Internet technology to deliver a behavioral weight loss program. *JAMA.* 2001;285:1172–1177
74. Downs J, Murray P, Bruine W, Penrose J, Palmgren C, Fischhoff B. Interactive video behavioral intervention to reduce adolescent females' STD risk: a randomized controlled trial. *Soc Sci Med.* 2004;59:1561–1572
75. Evers K, Prochaska JO, Van Marter D, Johnson J, Prochaska JM. Transtheoretical-based bullying prevention effectiveness trials in middle schools and high schools. *Educ Res.* 2007; In press

Adolesc Med 18 (2007) 400–406

Harnessing Technology for Adolescent Health Promotion

Paula M. Castaño, MD, MPH[a,*],
Raquel Andrés Martínez, PhD, MSc[a,b]

[a]*Department of Obstetrics and Gynecology, Columbia University Medical Center, 622 West 168th Street, New York, NY 10032, USA*

[b]*Centre for Research on Welfare Economics, Parc Científic de Barcelona, Campus Diagonal, University of Barcelona, Building D, Baldiri Reixac, 4–6, Floor 3, Suite B2, 08028 Barcelona, Spain*

V.L. is a 17-year-old presenting to an urban family-planning clinic for a pregnancy test. She had 1 previous pregnancy that ended in a miscarriage, after which she was prescribed birth control pills. She reports having a hard time remembering to take her pills and being confused about what to do when she misses one. On this visit, V.L. is seeking contraception. Despite comprehensive contraceptive counseling she is considering only birth control pills; she is afraid of the adverse effects of other contraceptive methods. She wants to finish high school and plans to study psychology in college. When asked when her last menstrual period was, she pulls out her cell phone and searches her wireless calendar.

Clinicians who care for sexually active adolescents commonly encounter stories like V.L.'s. Many US adolescents are sexually active, and most would be upset by a pregnancy. Most sexually active adolescents have tried contraceptives, but correct, consistent use is difficult to attain, and discontinuation rates are high, especially for birth control pills. There is no simple solution to improving contraceptive continuation, but there is large incentive. Contraceptive misuse results in unintended pregnancies that carry personal and societal repercussions. The most successful adolescent pregnancy-prevention programs have used innovative, multifactorial approaches. Here we describe a study that we are undertaking to evaluate a novel approach to improving contraceptive use by teens.

Our study involves daily cell-phone text-message contraceptive reminders. As with most novel technologies, younger generations are at the forefront of text

---

*Corresponding author.
E-mail address: pc2137@columbia.edu (P. M. Castaño).

messaging and cell-phone use. We have surveyed urban teens about their cell-phone use and text-messaging habits and will test whether text-message contraceptive reminders are a feasible means of improving contraceptive continuation and knowledge. We also foresee this simple technology being used as a delivery mechanism to remind adolescents about medication, appointments, and test results.

BACKGROUND

Sexual Activity in Adolescents

The National Survey of Family Growth is a periodic nationwide study that examines sexual activity, contraceptive use, and childbearing. The most recent 2002 survey revealed that 46% of all teens aged 15 to 19 have had intercourse, a decline from 55% in 1995.[1] Despite this decrease, 4.6 million teen girls remain at risk for pregnancy.[1] Sexually active teens who do not use birth control have a 90% chance of becoming pregnant in the following year.[2]

Contraceptive Use by Adolescents

Although 98% of sexually active teenaged girls have used a contraceptive method at some time,[1] only 82% were using a method at the time of the survey,[3] and only 75% used a method at first intercourse.[1] The percentage of black and Hispanic teens who used contraception was lower than white teens.[1] Among teens who used contraceptives, 53% used oral contraceptives (OCs), the highest percentage among all reproductive-aged groups.[3] OCs need to be used consistently to be effective.

Contraceptive Misuse and Discontinuation

In a study of OC use in inner-city family-planning clinics, Westhoff showed that women who rarely or never missed pills were more than twice as likely to continue OCs at 6 months than women who often missed pills. Discontinuation rates among the 595 teens were 53% and 75% at 3 and 6 months, respectively (Carolyn Westhoff, MD, Department of Obstetrics and Gynecology, Columbia University Medical Center, New York, NY, verbal communication, August 2006). Similar discontinuation rates have been reported elsewhere.[4-8] Teens discontinue OCs because they experience adverse effects, misunderstand instructions for use, and do not establish a pill-taking routine.[9] One million unintended pregnancies in the United States result from improper OC use, failure, or discontinuation.[10] In Westhoff's study, all but 1 of the pregnancies that did occur were in women who had discontinued their OCs during the study period.[11] Poor OC use by a teenager such as V.L. may result in an unintended pregnancy, a life-altering condition.

Adolescent Pregnancy and Its Consequences

In 2001, there were 80 pregnancies for every 1000 girls aged 15 to 19 in the United States.[12] More than 80% of the resulting 811 000 teen pregnancies were unintended.[13] According to the National Survey of Family Growth, the probability of a woman giving birth by the age of 20 is 18%. The probability rises to 35% for Hispanic women and 27% for black women.[1] Nationwide, the teenage pregnancy rate has dropped by 36% since its peak in 1990 but only by 19% in Hispanic teens.[12] New York State is ranked 14th in the nation for teen pregnancies, with 91 per 1000 teens becoming pregnant. For white New Yorkers, the teen pregnancy rate is only 52 per 1000, whereas the rates for Hispanic and black teens are 2½ to nearly 3½ times higher (130 and 167 per 1000, respectively).[12] In New York City, the teen pregnancy rate is 96 per 1000 teens, which is higher than the state and national rates.[14]

Unintended pregnancy has long-term consequences that can disproportionately affect teens. Pregnant teens are less likely to finish their education, more likely to be single parents, and less likely to acquire work experience, all factors that contribute to long-term decline in socioeconomic status.[15] Teen pregnancies are more likely to be medically complicated, with higher maternal and infant morbidity and mortality rates than those of older pregnant women.[15,16] More than one quarter of teen pregnancies end in abortion.[12] The effects of teen pregnancy can impact future generations, too; a daughter of a woman who gave birth in her teens is more likely to have a teen pregnancy herself.[1]

Cell Phones and Text Messaging

Pagers and timers have been used in the past for medication reminders. However, as technology has advanced, some tools have become much less popular. For example, new patients to our clinic are asked for contact information. In the past they often preferred being contacted via their home telephone and pager numbers. More recent contact sheets suggest that cell phones and e-mails are becoming much more widespread. Adolescents, in particular, are usually the first to adopt new technologies.

After seeing young patients use their cell phone for more than telephone calls, as V.L. did with her cell phone's calendar function, we considered the role that cell-phone text messaging could play in a clinical setting. Cell phones have recently become widespread in the United States, and cell-phone use continues to increase. A survey of wireless providers revealed that there were >219 million wireless subscribers in the United States in June 2006, nearly 50 million more than there were in the 2 previous years.[17] Nearly 50 billion text messages were sent in the last 6 months of 2005, which is double the amount from the previous year.[18] Sixty-four percent of teens with cell phones use text messaging, and urban teen girls are more likely to use text messaging than boys or adults.[19] Americans use cell phones for more than talking; they use text messaging to vote for reality-television contestants, receive daily jokes, and download ring tones.

Wireless text messaging has been used for longer and in greater numbers in other countries, where studies have evaluated its usefulness in clinical situations. Clinic reminders sent via text messages to parents increased clinic attendance by children and adolescents in Australia.[20] Text messaging was also found to be more effective than telephone callbacks and scheduled clinic revisits in providing patients in London, England, with chlamydia test results and decreasing the time it took for them to return to the clinic for treatment.[21] Text messaging was effective in improving medication adherence in clinical trials of vaccines and smoking cessation in Spain and South Africa.[22,23] However, it was not successful as part of a bulimia nervosa aftercare program in London.[24] There are no studies of the effectiveness of text-message reminders on contraceptive-continuation rates.

CASE STUDY: CAN YOU HEAR ME NOW?

To assess the use of technology in our population, we conducted a feasibility survey of 2521 racially diverse reproductive-aged women,[25] including 473 teens, who were attending 4 family-planning clinics in New York City. We collected limited demographic data in this anonymous survey. One of 4 sites for the survey contributed 58% of subjects. This partly Title X–funded, community-based clinic provided care to 2170 teens who made 4500 visits in 2005. Ninety-eight percent of the patients at this clinic were Hispanic or black, and 96% of the patients reported incomes below 100% of the federal poverty level. A second site contributed 33% of the subjects. This family-planning clinic provided care to 2500 racially diverse teens in 2005.

Our adolescent subjects ranged in age from 12 to 19 years. Only 3% chose to complete the survey in Spanish. Overall, 77% of the teens reported having a cell phone, and 89% of them reported being able to receive text messages. More than one third of the teens reported text-messaging at least once a day, and 54% rarely or never worried about the cost when text-messaging their friends. Only 11% of adolescents in this survey reported sharing their cell phone with someone else, and they had the same cell-phone number for an average of 0.8 years. One third of the participants in this feasibility survey worried about forgetting to take their medications,[25] and a similar proportion would like to receive text-message reminders for this. Given a choice between cell-phone calls, telephone calls, text messages, and e-mails as a means of receiving clinic-appointment reminders, 52% of the adolescents would choose cell-phone calls, and 26% would prefer text messages.

For now, V.L. decides to set a daily alarm in her cell phone as a reminder to take her pill. She also opts to receive a reminder for her next clinic appointment via a text message.

"TXT NOW 2 PREVENT PREGNANCIES L8R" STUDY PROPOSAL

Noting that cell-phone text-messaging use is nearly ubiquitous in an economically disadvantaged, young population, we designed a study to test the effectiveness of text-message reminders on contraceptive continuation. Our study takes advantage of this inexpensive, ubiquitous, and simple technology. We will use this technology to provide health information and personalized medication reminders in a novel and confidential way. The content of the messages will be geared toward teens and will incorporate the 10 characteristics of effective sex-education programs.[26] These characteristics include focusing on reducing behaviors that lead to teen pregnancy, reinforcing clear contraceptive messages, providing basic and accurate information, incorporating the culture of teens, and lasting a sufficient period of time.[26]

Our text messages address reasons for discontinuation by providing information about management of common OC adverse effects. They aim to aid teens in establishing a pill-taking routine by serving as a daily reminder for dosing. Finally, they provide information about common OC dosing problems (eg, what to do with missed pills) that teens may have forgotten since their screening visit.

We beta-tested the bilingual (English and Spanish) message-generating system with 10 OC users and made adjustments on the basis of the feedback we received. The text messages read: "Hi [subject name]. Remember to take your [name of birth control pill] today." Each reminder is accompanied by a short educational message that lists the benefits of contraceptive use and provides instructions for avoiding common medication errors. Alternately, teens can elect to receive entertaining text messages that contain their horoscope, celebrity news, sports news, or weather forecasts, further securing their confidentiality.

The study will take place in 2007–2008 at one of the urban family-planning clinics that served as a site for the initial pilot. We will randomly assign 960 teenagers who request OCs for birth control and compare the 6-month continuation rates in 480 teens who receive text-message reminders with 480 teens who receive routine care. Subjects will be able to customize the start date and time for text messages. Subjects will have an in-person baseline interview at enrollment and a follow-up telephone interview at the end of 6 cycles. At the baseline interview, subjects will answer questions about their previous contraceptive-use history, their reproductive history, their cell-phone use and text-messaging habits, and their baseline health knowledge. The interview will include questions concerning beliefs about adverse effects of hormonal contraception and what to do if OCs are misused.

At the follow-up visit we will ask each subject if she is currently using the pill and ascertain the subject's total duration of OC use since enrollment. If the subject discontinued the OCs, we will attempt to determine the reason(s). We will also ask questions regarding cell-phone and text-messaging habits, health knowledge, sexual activity to assess time at risk of pregnancy (relationship status, new contacts or relationships), and pregnancy and its outcome if it occurred during the study period.

Subjects will be compensated to help offset the cost of additional text-messaging use. The primary outcome of interest will be differences in continuation rates between the intervention and control groups at 6 months.

CONCLUSIONS

Teens are often at the forefront of technologic advances, and practitioners need to keep up with them. Text messaging can be used by clinicians to better care for their adolescent patients. The findings of this study could suggest novel ways to use text messaging to target more than contraceptive continuation. A similar approach could be applied to chronic illnesses for which medication adherence is key. Clinicians could consider confidentially text-messaging their patients regarding test results, medication refills, and upcoming clinic appointments. In the past, this required home telephone calls and mailings that could be intercepted.

Text messaging is a user-friendly technology that requires minimal data entry and willing users. This technology has the potential to benefit traditionally disadvantaged populations, reduce disparities, and increase access to health care services. Furthermore, as electronic health records become the standard for documentation, we need to explore integrating text-messaging capabilities with these systems.

REFERENCES

1. Abma JC, Martinez GM, Mosher WD, Dawson BS. Teenagers in the United States: sexual activity, contraceptive use, and childbearing, 2002. *Vital Health Stat 23*. 2004;(24):1–48
2. Harlap S, Kost K, Forrest JD. *Preventing Pregnancy, Protecting Health: A New Look at Birth Control Choices in the United States*. New York, NY: Alan Guttmacher Institute; 1991:36–37
3. Mosher WD, Martinez GM, Chandra A, Abma JC, Wilson SJ. Use of contraception and use of family planning services in the United States: 1982–2002. *Adv Data*. 2004;(350):1–36
4. Emans SJ, Grace E, Woods ER, Smith DE, Klein K, Merola J. Adolescents' compliance with the use of oral contraceptives. *JAMA*. 1987;257:3377–3381
5. Furstenberg FF Jr, Shea J, Allison P, Herceg-Baron R, Webb D. Contraceptive continuation among adolescents attending family planning clinics. *Fam Plann Perspect*. 1983;15:211–214, 216–217
6. Glei DA. Measuring contraceptive use patterns among teenage and adult women. *Fam Plann Perspect*. 1999;31:73–80
7. Trussell J, Vaughan B. Contraceptive failure, method-related discontinuation and resumption of use: results from the 1995 National Survey of Family Growth. *Fam Plann Perspect*. 1999;31:64–72, 93
8. Zibners A, Cromer BA, Hayes J. Comparison of continuation rates for hormonal contraception among adolescents. *J Pediatr Adolesc Gynecol*. 1999;12:90–94
9. Rosenberg MJ, Waugh MS, Meehan TE. Use and misuse of oral contraceptives: risk indicators for poor pill taking and discontinuation. *Contraception*. 1995;51:283–288

. Rosenberg MJ, Waugh MS, Long S. Unintended pregnancies and use, misuse and discontinuation of oral contraceptives. *J Reprod Med.* 1995;40:355–360

11. Westhoff C, Heartwell S, Edwards S, et al. Initiation of oral contraceptives using a quick start compared with a conventional start: a randomized, controlled trial. *Obstet Gynecol.* 2007;109: 1270–1276

12. Guttmacher Institute. U.S. teenage pregnancy statistics: national and state trends and trends by race and ethnicity. Available at: www.guttmacher.org/pubs/2006/09/12/USTPstats.pdf. Accessed March 4, 2007

13. Finer LB, Henshaw SK. Disparities in rates of unintended pregnancy in the United States, 1994 and 2001. *Perspect Sex Reprod Health.* 2006;38:90–96

14. New York State Department of Health. Table 30: total pregnancies and teenage pregnancies by type and resident county page. Available at: www.health.state.ny.us/nysdoh/vital_statistics/2004/table30.htm. Accessed March 4, 2007

15. Brown SS, Eisenberg L, eds. *The Best Intentions: Unintended Pregnancy and the Well-being of Children and Families.* Washington, DC: National Academy Press; 1995:55–59

16. Klein JD; American Academy of Pediatrics, Committee on Adolescence. Adolescent pregnancy: current trends and issues. *Pediatrics.* 2005;116:281–286

17. CTIA. Background on CTIA's semi-annual wireless industry survey. Available at: http://files.ctia.org/pdf/CTIAMidYear2006Survey.pdf. Accessed February 13, 2007

18. Wireless Telecommunications Bureau. Eleventh annual report and analysis of competitive market conditions with respect to commercial mobile services. Available at: http://hraunfoss.fcc.gov/edocs_public/attachmatch/FCC-06-142A1.pdf. Accessed March 4, 2007

19. Lenhart A, Madden M, Hitlin P. Pew Internet & American Life Project: teens and technology—youth are leading the transition to a fully wired and mobile nation. Available at: www.pewinternet.org/pdfs/PIP_Teens_Tech_July2005web.pdf. Accessed March 30, 2006

20. Downer SR, Meara JG, Da Costa AC, Sethuraman K. SMS text messaging improves outpatient attendance. *Aust Health Rev.* 2006;30:389–396

21. Menon-Johansson AS, McNaught F, Mandalia S, Sullivan AK. Texting decreases the time to treatment for genital *Chlamydia trachomatis* infection. *Sex Transm Infect.* 2006;82:49–51

22. Vilella A, Bayas J, Diaz M, et al. The role of mobile phones in improving vaccination rates in travelers. *Prev Med.* 2004;38:503–509

23. Rodgers A, Corbett T, Bramley D, et al. Do u smoke after txt? Results of a randomized trial of smoking cessation using mobile phone text messaging. *Tob Control.* 2005;14:255–261

24. Robinson S, Perkins S, Bauer S, Hammond N, Treasure J, Schmidt U. Aftercare intervention through text messaging in the treatment of bulimia nervosa: feasibility pilot. *Int J Eat Disord.* 2006;39:633–638

25. Castaño PM, Andres R, Lara M, Westhoff C. Assessing feasibility of text messaging to improve medication adherence. *Obstet Gynecol.* 2006;107(suppl):40S

26. Kirby D. *Emerging Answers: Research Findings on Programs to Reduce Teen Pregnancy (Summary).* Washington, DC: National Campaign to Prevent Teen Pregnancy; 2001:10

Adolesc Med 18 (2007) 407–414

Health Information for Young People Where and When They Most Want It: A Case Study of www.teenagehealthfreak.org

Ann McPherson[a],*, CBE, MB, BS, FRCGP, DCH,
Aidan Macfarlane, FRCP, FRCPCH, FFPH[b]

[a]Department of Public Health and Primary Care, University of Oxford, Old Road, Headington OX3 LF, United Kingdom

[b]Independent Consultant, 6 Cobden Crescent, Oxford OX1 4LJ, United Kingdom

The www.teenagehealthfreak.org Web site was developed in response to the popularity of a pair of youth-oriented books we published in 1989 and 1990. *The Diary of a Teenage Health Freak*[1] and *I'm a Health Freak, Too*[2] were written to address a recognizable absence of health-related information designed for teenagers. The books have sold >1 million copies domestically thus far and have been translated into 23 different languages for distribution globally.

In less than a decade's time, the information in the books seemed limited by the paper-bound nature of its publication. The rapid development of the Internet in the 1990s provided an opportunity to present the many sexual and reproductive health facts contained within them in a more interactive and accessible format. After receiving the financial backing of a business philanthropist, we established www.teenagehealthfreak.org based on the now commonly accepted understanding that young people are simultaneously interested in both immediate information that respects their sexual decision-making process and new technologies that enhance their lives.

In its current form, the Web site was designed to provide adolescents with accessible, evidence-based information on health-related matters that contextually fit their everyday lives. The material is meant to complement rather than substitute presently available sources of health information for young people. For example, we do not intend to replace health practitioners or educators but, instead, enhance their work with an accessible, timely resource.

*Corresponding author.
E-mail address: ann.mcpherson@dphpc.ox.ac.uk (A. McPherson).

During development, we decided on several characteristics that we felt were critical to a successful online experience. The site needed to be free of all advertising, remain as evidence based as possible, align itself with the key stages of the government's education strategy, and remain largely interactive. Intrinsic in the process of determining our prerequisites was a need to balance our design with the strict confidentiality regulations stipulated in the United Kingdom Data Protection Act. Although in most instances these choices helped popularize www.teenagehealthfreak.org, some of our decisions (particularly remaining free of advertising) became an impediment in building a sustainable Web-based resource.

During development we sought the opinions of our target audience to help construct the site in ways that they deemed helpful. Several Internet-based focus groups of young people made content and semantic suggestions. Their input was crucial to our success, and because of this, we initiated a system that allows constant feedback from the youth who are accessing the site, akin to that provided by our early focus groups. Feedback from adolescents is used to create a dynamic environment that reflects the interests and needs of those who seek its information. We believe, in the end, that we were able to construct a site that deals with all aspects of young people's lives, not just those that are medical. The focus on simple, dynamic content (avoiding lengthy downloads and advertisements) ultimately made the site more accessible.

We launched the site in 2000 and almost immediately alerted all personal and social health education teachers by mail with the hope that they would introduce the site in their classrooms. Similarly, we sent government-sponsored leaflets to adolescent clinical practitioners and their patients. This information campaign was largely successful. www.teenagehealthfreak.org has remained in the top 5 sites searched for on Google under the term "teenage health." It has sustained an average of 1.5 million hits per month since its inception. In addition, the Web site won the British United Provident Association (BUPA) Communication award in 2001 for excellence in medical research and health care. Currently, site content is provided by us.

CONTENT

The Web site itself is divided into 2 parts: "Teenage Health Freak" and "Dr Anne's Virtual Surgery." Both sites can be accessed via the homepage (www-.teenagehealthfreak.org), but the virtual clinic (a simulated adolescent health clinic) is also directly available at www.drann.org.

Teenage Health Freak

This portion of the site contains the online diary (written by us) of a fictitious 15-year-old teenager, Pete Payne. Pete updates his diary daily with his worries and traumas plus those of his family and friends. Pete has discovered Dr Ann's site, and his diary often links to it for information on his latest health worry. Pete's diary is a humorous, teenage-friendly, relevant health-information resource designed to encourage visitors to return and keep up-to-date with events in his life. Here is an example:

My diary for Monday, 22/01/2007

Monday. Awake most of last night. At 1 a.m. decided that it was still on with Cills, 2 a.m. it was off, 3 a.m. it was on again, 4.12 a.m. it was off 4 good. This morning still off, so finally emailed her when I dragged meself out of bed saying,

"Dear Cills, thanks 4 your email. I'm the nicest boy that I know 2, but I can't go 4 this 'on-off' business. 2 wearing on me hormones. So it's off 4 good this time—sorry—you never really was a girlfriend. Pete"

And that was it, 'cept I immediately wanted her back again once I'd sent it. Wonder if there is a *legal age* at which one can chuck one's first girlfriend? Did I do right peeps?

Key words in the diary relating to health issues such as "acne," "depression," "sex," and, as seen above, "legal age" along with hundreds of other health concerns are linked to Dr Ann's clinic. We continuously update the diary to include relevant events from around the world, especially those relating to health issues.

Dr Ann's Virtual Surgery

This is the virtual adolescent clinic of Pete's doctor. The site is full of medical information about common teenage health worries phrased in a manner that is both age appropriate and accessible. Central is an index of >300 words, many of which include slang terms as well as the appropriate medical terminology. We have focused on mental and emotional health concerns in addition to physical ailments (eg, entries under "A" include "abortion," "addiction," "age and legal rights," "anger," "anorexia nervosa," "anxiety," and "attention deficit disorder").

The clinic itself is split into 8 main sections, each of which focuses on separate topical categories: (1) emergency department; (2) not feeling well (general health concerns); (3) drugs and alcohol; (4) sex; (5) smoking; (6) weight and eating; (7) moods; and (8) body changes. The last category is separated into specifications for boys and girls. Additional sections include quizzes and surveys, a notice board for general health advice, and a series of external links to other useful health sites. These additional sections create a dynamic atmosphere in which youth can engage particular topics in greater depth. Questionnaires in particular unassumingly solicit youth to question their own health behavior under topics titled "What stresses you out?" and "RU the right W8?"

Key to Dr Ann's clinic is an e-mail exchange facility where teenagers can contact the doctor in confidence with their own health problems via the "ask Dr Ann" option. Although it is clearly stated on the site that Dr Ann cannot respond to all questions, new key questions and answers appear daily.

The process for e-mails is as follows:

1. E-mails are automatically scanned for keywords that appear in the site's index. If a keyword is found, the person corresponding is e-mailed back with a recommendation of where they should look for more information on the Web site.
2. All identifying data (name, demographics, etc) are then removed (per United Kingdom Data Protection Act mandates), and the e-mail is stored in a separate site-management system.
3. The separate "site-management" store of past e-mails is regularly reviewed by one of the authors, and e-mails of particular relevance are answered. The question and response are posted on the site. One new e-mail correspondence is posted each day.
4. The bulk of the e-mails are, at regular intervals, analyzed for content and classified into 1 of 23 main categories. Additional details of e-mail analysis are outlined in Tables 1–3.

OBSTACLES

Since establishing the Web site there have been a number of problems. Ascertaining the logistics behind national advertising was difficult. We needed to discover an easy, cost-effective way to make large amounts of people aware of the site quickly. To do this, we tried 2 means. First, we sent suggestions on how to use the site as a classroom tool to all relevant teachers throughout the United Kingdom. Second, we capitalized on the "up-front" sexual health content to attract broadcast and print media. The combined effect of these 2 methods drew traffic to our site that generated a much-needed "word-of-mouth" profile.

Our second major hurdle came from structures established for information technology within schools. Basically, our site was blocked by filters that prevented youth from accessing sites with explicit sexual content. Although our site displays only sexual health information (rather than pictures or other media), we were censored similar to pornography. In response, we contacted the companies responsible for managing the school servers and explained exactly what our site was trying to achieve. With some persistence, we were able to have our site removed from the filter.

Finally, as alluded to earlier, our unstable finances for maintaining the site have been difficult to overcome. Without advertising we have turned to philanthropic and governmental support. A grant from the English government is currently our largest source of support. A more long-term strategy will need to be identified.

ASSESSING www.teenagehealthfreak.org

Confidentiality laws in the United Kingdom combined with the general reluctance on the part of our target audience to attach identifying information to sensitive material make assessing the exact demographics of our site's users difficult. Our developmental focus groups advised us that most young people would not want to access the site if identifying information was required. This has necessitated relying on data for analysis that may be subject to serious inaccuracies. The most readily available source for data are the e-mails sent by site users.

Currently, ~50 000 e-mails are received from young people each year, with a total of ~250 000 since we started. These e-mails indicate that the main age group of those using the site is 14-year-olds (range: 10–17 years). We conducted an analysis of 28 634 e-mails received between January 1 and December 31, 2003. Although we recognize the large margin of error that may exist in this analysis, our discussion below presumes that these e-mails are indicative of the larger population of e-mail senders.

Girls e-mail more than boys in an approximate ratio of 2:1. Of these, 27% ($n = 7731$) were impossible to answer for various reasons. Tables 1 through 3 contain relevant analysis of these e-mails.

The high proportion of e-mails with questions about sexuality is not an unexpected finding (Table 1). Girls were more likely than boys to query the site for information on relationship issues and concerns about body image. We believe the inconsistent nature of sex education in the United Kingdom combined with the hypersensitivity toward sex experienced during adolescence contributes greatly to the number of sexuality-focused questions.

When examining a specific question regarding sexuality (Table 2), girls overwhelmingly inquired about pregnancy (eg, "What is the chance of getting pregnant if you use a condom?"), whereas many boys focused on their genitalia (eg, "I have white spots on my penis, is that normal?"). Alternatively, we did

Table 1
Topics of e-mails

	Boys, n	Girls, n	Unknown, n	Overall, N
Sex	42	48	10%	53
Drugs	31	60	9	17
Body image	18	74	8	12
Illness	23	64	13	9
Relationships	28	62	10	7
Other	—	—	—	2

Table 2
Analysis of e-mails about sex according to subcategory (N = 11 272)

Subcategory	Boys, %	Girls, %	Unknown, %	Overall, %
Serious, sexual	35	55	10	40
Serious, penis	86	6	8	17
Pregnancy	15	77	8	12
Gender issues	54	37	9	8
Menstruation	3	90	7	8
Sexual nonsense	66	23	11	7
Puberty	46	46	6	8

receive a number of e-mails that were considered nonsense, especially from boys (eg, "My penis is 3 foot long will I hurt my girlfriend?").

Finally, as can be seen in Table 3, we received a range of "illness" concerns that our users may have felt were too basic or too sensitive to ask their health provider. For example, we received a large number of questions from girls regarding mood (eg, "I really feel like killing myself—please help me") and fatigue (eg, "I am always tired"). Boys were less likely to ask about illness than girls.

CONCLUSIONS: FUTURE DEVELOPMENT

There are a number of specific developments of the www.teenagehealthfreak.org Web site that will be undertaken in the near future.

Links to www.youthhealthtalk.org

This Web site is part of a data base of individual patient experiences (www.d-ipex.org). It is based on qualitative research using videotaped interviews that examine youth experience of health and illness such as early sexual experience and cancer. Approximately 40 young people are interviewed for each health issue to provide a wide range of experiences that reflect socioeconomic, racial, and

Table 3
Analysis of e-mails about illness according to subcategory (N = 1964)

Subcategory	Boys, %	Girls, %	Unknown, %	Overall, %
Moods	19	73	8	29
Skin problems	26	63	11	29
Minor illnesses	26	62	12	21
Serious illnesses	27	53	20	16
Fatigue	23	71	6	3

gender differences. The future proposal is to link www.teenagehealthfreak.org and www.youthhealthtalk.org in such a way that the former would initiate the discussion of certain health topics for youth, whereas the latter would go more in depth and provide social and biographical information related to disease.

Universal Health Questionnaire

The Department of Health in England is piloting a universal health questionnaire for all 10- to 14-year-olds throughout the country on the www.teenagehealth-freak.org Web site. The responses are confidential, but depending on individual answers, the participating youth will be referred electronically to a number of different Web sites that provide additional health-related information and services. Questions that are raised within the context of the survey are handled in the same manner that e-mails to Dr Ann are handled. Financing is provided by the English Department of Health.

Accelerated Correspondence

Funding has been obtained to increase the number of e-mails that can be answered per week from 5 to 40. Ways in which the answers to these e-mails can still be posted on the site but also sent directly to the young person answering them, without infringing on the United Kingdom Data Protection Act, are being examined.

Other Developments

Funding is being sought to develop (1) a "search" function for the site that would allow youth to access more nuanced information quickly, (2) systems that continuously update content- and time-specific elements of the site on a regular basis, (3) more quizzes, (4) a site-manager system that would allow us to make content adjustments directly rather than through the site's managing company, and (5) systems that provide youth with more self-management skills.

Editor's note: www.teenagehealthfreak.org is a United Kingdom–based Web site designed to provide younger adolescents with direct, easy-to-access health information. Drs Macfarlane and McPherson developed the site (and the books that preceded it) in response to adolescent needs they discovered in their clinical practices. Dr Macfarlane previously ran the child and adolescent health services for Oxfordshire, England, and now works as an independent consultant in the strategic planning of child and adolescent health services. Dr McPherson is a family doctor and lecturer practicing in Oxford.

www.teenagehealthfreak.org is not intended as a behavioral intervention but, rather, a resource for youth in search of reliable, unbiased information. Although the case study discussed is context specific to the United Kingdom, it is meant as a model for other Internet-based health initiatives and as a demonstration of early adolescent health information on the Internet.

REFERENCES

1. Macfarlane A, McPherson A. *The Diary of a Teenage Health Freak.* London, United Kingdom: Oxford Paperbacks; 1987
2. Macfarlane A, McPherson A. *I Am a Health Freak, Too.* London, United Kingdom: Oxford Paperbacks; 1989

Adolesc Med 18 (2007) 415–424

One Chip at a Time: Using Technology to Enhance Youth Development

Alwyn Cohall, MD*, Montsine Nshom, MPH, Andrea Nye, MPH

Harlem Health Promotion Center, Columbia University Mailman School of Public Health, 215 West 125th Street, Ground Floor, New York, NY 10027, USA

The concept of youth development has garnered considerable attention recently because of its potential to reduce or prevent high-risk problem behaviors.[1] Defined as the level of comfort and confidence that youth associate with their emotional, psychological, and social transition into adulthood, youth development is a guiding principle of many youth service programs.[2] These programs often use a number of strategies to engage and retain youth, including community service and outreach or general mentoring.[3] Likewise, education and training on specific subject matters, such as music or sports, have also been commonly used as a "hook" to attract youth. Recently, technology has also surfaced as another important content area.

Given young people's natural inclination toward the use of technology, youth development programs are embracing this as a tool to attract and retain participation while promoting healthy adolescent development and increasing technologic literacy. Therefore, the purpose of this article is to provide a brief overview of the intersection between youth development and technology and illustrate the potential for this approach to assist youth in transforming their lives.

YOUTH DEVELOPMENT

Youth development is defined as the level of comfort and confidence that youth associate with skills and competencies needed in their emotional, psychological, and social transition into adulthood.[2] Most young people undergo the process of development among their family and peers, as well as within their school, neighborhood, and community settings. For some, this can be a challenging time. Marked with exploration and experimentation, adolescents often engage in high-risk behaviors including substance use, unsafe sex, and reckless driving. Simi-

*Corresponding author.
E-mail address: atc1@columbia.edu (A. Cohall).

larly, factors such as race, gender, socioeconomic status, and sexual orientation play an important role in psychological and social development, especially if the adolescent is a member of a minority group.[4] The challenges associated with adolescence can be amplified for those who find themselves marginalized or even rejected by family, friends, and society at large. However, research has shown that when given opportunities to participate in their communities in meaningful ways, young people not only can gain a sense of civic duty and enhanced connection to the community but also report increased self-esteem and enhanced leadership skills.[5]

OVERVIEW OF YOUTH DEVELOPMENT PROGRAMS

Youth development programs are created to meet developmental needs by providing an environment in which young people can build and master the competencies and skills that are necessary for successful transition into adulthood.[6] These programs emphasize personal and social development and encourage engagement in the community, positive self-image, and competency building among youth.[2] Along with personal growth and development, many programs also promote physical health and well-being by integrating health promotion and wellness into their goals and objectives.[7] Overall, youth development programs attempt to offer unique challenges, experiences, and learning opportunities that are aimed at helping youth reach their full potential.[8]

Programs use a variety of frameworks, each with a slightly different approach. For example, whereas the Search Institute highlights internal and external developmental asset building with the help of friends, family, and peers,[9] the Community Action Framework by Connell and Gambone[10] emphasizes a top-down approach for setting long-term goals for young people and then encourages community stakeholders to facilitate the tasks necessary to achieve those goals. Similarly, other programs use a resiliency framework that is aimed at surrounding youth with positive, caring adults who have high expectations and can help participants mature in the face of adversity.[11] More specifically, one resiliency-based, pro–civic participation framework is the Youth Development Model.[2] This model emphasizes personal development, social development, and community engagement, be it through sports, vocational training, or other activities.[2] The model also promotes the 5 core assets of effective positive youth development programs: confidence, character, connections, competence, and caring.[8]

Regardless of the approach, however, programs dedicated to youth development have a similar goal: to help young people become healthy, successful adults through a concerted effort to provide primary or secondary prevention and promote positive behavior.[1] Effective programs welcome and value diversity in both their participants and their services. Furthermore, they allow youth to connect to adults in a positive setting while providing a safe space for personal growth, health, and wellness.[1] Although some programs focus on sports and fitness, others address these issues by focusing on correlated topics such as the visual or dramatic arts. There are a number of methods and tools available; one such tool that is increasingly common is the use of technology.

YOUTH AND TECHNOLOGY

Over the years, young people have consistently shown themselves to be avid users of technology. Lenhart et al[12] reported that in the United States, ~87% of young people aged 12 to 17 use the Internet, up 14% from 2000; this is in comparison to 66% of adult US Internet users.[12] The most common tasks performed online by young people include sending and receiving e-mail, visiting Web sites for information on popular culture, playing games, getting news on current events, and sending or receiving instant messages.[12] In information seeking, 50% of all adolescent Internet users and 44% of urban female adolescent Internet users report using the Internet to seek out information on diet, exercise, or sexual-health–related issues such as birth control or sexually transmitted infections.[13–15] As can be seen, a majority of activities are aimed at extending and sustaining social networks and accessing health information.[16]

Along with extending social networks and enhancing access to information, technology can also play an essential role in building self-esteem and improving self-efficacy around technologic literacy. Information technology provides an immense opportunity for youth development.[17] Research has shown that youth who have access to technology have increased self-esteem, higher educational levels, and better socioeconomic prospects than their counterparts who do not use technology. For example, Valaitis[18] found that young people's perceptions of technology were positive and empowering. Participants involved in a school-based community development project felt that learning and mastering technology decreased their social anxiety toward working and communicating with adults and increased their sense of self and control over their surroundings. Those who were surveyed also reported increased opportunities for self-reflection and decision-making, 2 of many developmental assets that are key to positive youth development.[18] Similarly, technology used as a tool within youth development programs can provide a social setting for group interactions, thus allowing room for enhanced interpersonal relationships and skill building.[18]

A number of youth development programs nationwide make technology a cornerstone of their organizations. For example, more than 100 Intel Computer Clubhouses worldwide provide after-school learning environments for urban youth to explore their interests through computers and technology. Similar programs can be found from California (Eastmont Computing Center of Oakland and Bayview Hunter's Point Center for Arts and Technology) to New York (Harlem Congregation for Community Improvement's Computer Clubhouse). Other organizations, such as ReelGirls and Evergreen Youth Television in Washington State, Teen Voices in Boston, Massachusetts, and VOX Teen Communications in Atlanta, Georgia, focus on media and film technology. These organizations combine mentorship and technologic advancement in an attempt to facilitate both personal and professional growth.

TECHNOLOGY AND YOUTH DEVELOPMENT: BRIDGING THE GAP

Despite the presence of many successful and innovative programs, a gap still exists between technology "haves" and "have-nots." This digital divide continues to keep certain groups from benefiting from the growing trends and opportunities associated with technology and the Internet. According to Lenhart et al,[12] 13% of US teenagers have yet to use the Internet; a majority of these youth are limited by socioeconomic status.[19,20] More often than not, these youth are black or Hispanic. In fact, it is estimated that 73% of teens in families with incomes of $30 000 or less are online (in comparison to 90% of teens from families with incomes of $50 000 or more).[12] Thus, teens who are marginalized by race tend to be marginalized from access to technology and technologic literacy as well.[21,22]

Given the link between technologic literacy, academic achievement, and future socioeconomic and health status, it becomes apparent that at-risk, minority youth could greatly benefit from programs that use technology as a tool for youth development.[18,22] Not only would young people who participate in these programs increase their access to technology and technologic literacy, but they would also have the opportunity to gain the skills and competencies that lead to healthy adolescent development.[8]

TECHNOLOGY AS A TOOL FOR YOUTH DEVELOPMENT: 2 CASE STUDIES

The following case studies focus on 2 programs that provide services for youth residing in the community of Harlem in New York City. A historical area of New York, Harlem has seen as much advancement as it has adversity in the last few decades. This community has nurtured the development of many famous musicians, artists, athletes, political advocates, and religious leaders; however, it has also been a community historically beset by a number of significant problems. For example, a landmark study released by McCord and Freeman[23] in 1990 noted that the average life span of black men residing in Harlem was less than men who live in some developing countries.

Over the past 10 years, significant changes have occurred within the Harlem community. Designated as one the nation's federal empowerment zones, several large businesses have moved into the community, thus boosting the local economy. Similarly, faith-based institutions, local, state, and federal agencies, and community-based organizations have begun to revitalize Harlem's crumbling housing infrastructure and create focused efforts on health-improvement initiatives. Much additional work is needed.

As in many marginalized communities, youth living in Harlem often find themselves walking a narrow tightrope as they seek to make healthy transitions into adulthood. Those who are successful often point to strong family support, dedicated schools, and community-based programs such as those outlined below as being instrumental to their success.

Given the community need and the potential for youth development programs to assist urban, minority, at-risk youth in health transitions, we were particularly interested in identifying programs that could convincingly demonstrate the successful use of technology as the basis for youth development programming. We focused on HarlemLive, an Internet publication that is produced for and maintained by young people, and Lehman Brothers Health Promotion Learning Lab (HPLL)† at the Harlem Children's Zone Promise Academy charter school. Both sites allowed us to visit their space and interview adults and youth in person, which provided an opportunity to observe the programs directly and hear participant and staff opinions.

HarlemLive is a nonprofit organization that is at once a media, technology, and leadership program that allows youth to work in all positions (from field journalists to producers, video photographers to video editors and editor-in-chief) related to the Web site. Participants learn through experience and thus receive an opportunity to gain specific skills and competencies in interpersonal and mass communications, leadership, and teamwork. The youth and staff involved with HarlemLive have received numerous awards and recognition for their work from sources such as Yahoo, Fleet Bank, and the New York Times.

The HPLL is located within Promise Academy, a charter school developed by the Harlem Children's Zone. The HPLL facilitates health promotion and technologic resourcefulness by engaging youth in culturally competent, age-appropriate, computer-based tours and activities that focus on health. Frequently used Web sites are BrainPop (www.brainpop.com), KidsHealth (www.kidshealth.org), and GoogleEarth (http://earth.google.com). Based on a peer-education model, high school student interns ("explainers") research, plan, and facilitate topics of interest for lesson plans and activities and then teach and mentor the Harlem Children's Zone Promise Academy students who visit HPLL. In turn, the explainers are taught and mentored by HPLL staff. The overall mission of the HPLL is to improve the health literacy of Harlem residents and, in turn, their overall health maintenance and status.

---

†The HPLL is a program of the Harlem Children's Health Project, funded by the Children's Health Fund.

Young people between the ages of 16 and 24 years were interviewed at both sites. Staff members who play integral roles in the day-to-day functioning of each program were interviewed as well. Interviews attempted to capture the past and current experiences with technology, perceived growth and development (both technologic and personal), and interpretations and thoughts on youth development in general. In visiting both sites, we found it encouraging that many of the reflections and stories paralleled the 5 "Cs" of the Youth Development Model: confidence, character, connections, competence, and caring.[8] Therefore, we have framed each case study with examples of these competencies and feature stories, quotes, and general reflections that clearly illustrate the positive outcomes associated with these programs.

Confidence

Confidence can be defined as one's overall sense of self-worth and level of self-esteem.[4,8] Mastering any skill can have a profound impact on a youth's sense of self-worth; technologic skills are no exception to this phenomenon. In fact, M.S., a video editor and journalist at HarlemLive, articulated his feelings of self-worth and esteem as he described how mastering a video-editing program changed they way he saw himself and others. He explained how he went from feeling anxious to adept: "I thought it would be impossible to learn. . .but then I thought, you know what, I'm gonna go hard on this. . .when you use these [technologies], it's like you have some sort of power. . .when you learn the stuff, you feel like you can do anything you want. . .like [you] have an advantage over other people."

Competence

Competence is characterized as one's self-efficacy in specific skill areas, be it social, academic, vocational, or otherwise.[4,8] Although most of the youth interviewed had basic computer skills and familiarity with general programs such as Microsoft Office and Internet Explorer before they started each program, few had experience with the task-specific programs they would soon master at each site. E.V., an explainer at the HPLL, described her initial feelings toward technology as anxious and fearful. This changed as she learned more about the programs and skills she was responsible for teaching to other students: "[There are] so many different things that I know how to do now that I actually didn't know before. And that I didn't want to try to because. . .when you don't know something, you don't want to do it because you feel like you're stupid because you don't know it." Her reflection illustrates the initial fear many youth may have about technology in general and how overcoming that fear helps one increase self-efficacy for specific skill sets. This, in turn, can translate into increased self-confidence and self-worth.

Character

Character is defined as a respect for right and wrong and the personality traits and characteristics that help individuals to make these distinctions.[4,8] We asked youth what skills, traits, or qualities they gained from their interactions with peers and adults at the programs in which they participated. Overwhelmingly positive responses included patience, time management, creative problem solving, and self-confidence, all of which are crucial for taking on the challenges that come with pending adulthood. HarlemLive's office manager noted that at HarlemLive, "we try to build leaders in our organization, so we give them a huge responsi-bility. . .keys to the space. . .money to buy stuff for the office. . .." R.C., the executive director of HarlemLive, supports this, stating that ". . .it's about own-ership. We make them responsible. They have to be accountable. [It's] become a big tenet of the program." Thus, at HarlemLive, youth develop character by being entrusted with not only the content of the online magazine itself but also the office responsibilities that go along with producing an online magazine.

At the HPLL, the explainers reflected on the characteristics gained from the peer-education model, explaining that they feel they are in unique position to both benefit from adult mentoring and serve as role models for younger students. As one explainer stated: "If I make a mistake, they'll let me know about it and they'll let me know about it very nicely. . . If they tell me I have to step up, I step up."

Connections

Connections can be defined as positive, strong bonds with both individuals and institutions, be they family, friends, school, work, or society at large.[4,8] We asked participants how they felt technology uniquely facilitated youth development and community engagement. The editor-in-chief at HarlemLive explained that the close proximity to the neighborhood makes participants more invested in their community: "Because HarlemLive is located in the middle of Harlem, we can just go out and look at our relatives and our neighbors, people in our commu-nity. . ... [T]hat brings us closer to the community because we work in the community." This connectedness to Harlem no doubt influences the stories and events that the journalists cover.

Similarly, the program director of the Harlem Children's Health Project, which oversees the HPLL, noted that the computer laboratory is merely the vessel in the journey toward community-based health advocacy. When asked about the ben-efits of technology as a tool for youth development, he noted that in comparison to sports or other similar activities, technology could be more applicable to each youth's future regardless of the direction they choose. He also highlighted the ability that technology has to link youth with external places and people they might not otherwise see or know, thus improving their interest in and ability to connect to Harlem and the world beyond.

Caring

Caring can be defined as the level of empathy or sympathy one has for others and one feels from others in return.[4,8] We inquired about the type of interactions that youth have with adults at their community-based organization and how, if at all, these experiences have changed the way youth view and interact with other adults in their lives. As an adult in his mid-20s, the office manager at HarlemLive falls between the youth and adult range of the age spectrum. He feels that this improves his ability to connect with the youth at HarlemLive, stating: "[L]ots of people come to me when they need help or they have something they need my advice for. . .." He described the relationships at HarlemLive as "family— because we do everything a family does. We hang out, we fight, we argue, we have fun. . ... [O]ur relationship goes outside the office." This level of caring not only affects the way youth relate to each other at HarlemLive but also the way they relate to others outside of the community-based organization. Development of empathy is not only an important milestone in adolescent development, it is also a journalistic skill that is needed to successfully understand community issues and develop relevant publications. Given their experiences with Harlem-Live, youth have no shortage of opportunities to care.

In the same way, one explainer at the HPLL explained that the adults with whom he works care about him beyond typical employee-employer–related interactions: "If something is wrong and it looks like something is wrong, [they will] ask you if something's wrong. . ... [T]hat brings out the best in us, and we are willing to work harder." Another explainer affirms this, stating: "If you tell them something, they're not judgmental, they will give their opinion to help you or give you advice but they won't judge you." Developing this level of trust and reliance with adults has, in some cases, shown youth a more positive side of authority figures and may influence their future relationships. In addition, compassion from staff members influences them to invest the same level of caring into the younger students who visit the learning laboratory.

Participant Definitions of Youth Development

Finally, we asked both the youth and adults at each community-based organization how they define youth development and what they felt were the components of an effective youth development program. Their answers were broad and diverse. Rather than synthesize these responses, the following are some thoughts from participants as a testament to what these programs strive to accomplish.

"Youth development is. . ."
- a "young [person] doing something to better themselves. . .doing something positive." (M.S., HarlemLive)
- "taking youth off the corners and off the streets. . .and putting them into organizations such as HarlemLive. . .to push these kids into doing something successful with their lives." (S.R., HarlemLive)

- "people, just the kids my age, younger than me probably, just trying to do good and try to grow up to be something successful, as opposed to everybody, adults and people looking down on us and thinking that because we're young we can't do as much." (E.V., HPLL)
- when "you learn how to go from a kid to being more of a young adult. And I think youth development not only involves. . .personal issues like self-image and all those types of stuff that goes into puberty and all that stuff, but more of how you view the world." (M.G., HPLL)
- "enlightenment, empowerment [and] self-awareness. It's growth. . .an opportunity for students to reach their potential, meet their potential, exceed potential. It is an opportunity to learn about options." (L.S., HPLL)

CONCLUSIONS

Research has shown that youth who have high connectedness to family, school, and their community are less likely to engage in risk-taking behaviors such as tobacco, alcohol, and substance use, interpersonal violence, and self-harm.[24,25] In response, youth development programs provide the opportunity to enhance personal and social development while also emphasizing community connections, positive self-image, and health and wellness overall. Technology-centered programs offer a compelling premise for engaging youth in efforts to increase technologic literacy, self-worth, and personal development.

Despite the apparent constructive qualities of these programs, formal evaluation should take place. If proven successful, there is ample opportunity to enhance positive outcomes by replicating these promising programs. From our experiences with HarlemLive and the HPLL, we feel that similar technology-based youth development programs have the potential to provide a lasting, constructive impact on youth who are making the transition to adulthood in our increasingly connected, changing, and fast-paced world.

ACKNOWLEDGMENTS

This work was supported by Centers for Disease Control and Prevention grant U48-DP000030.

Many thanks go to the HPLL and Harlem Children's Health Project staff, as well as its sponsor, the Children's Health Fund, for support and collaboration. We also thank the staff of HarlemLive for support and involvement in this article.

REFERENCES

1. Lerner R, Thomson LS. Promoting healthy adolescent behavior and development: issues in the design and evaluation of effective youth programs. *J Pediatr Nurs.* 2002;17:338–344
2. Greenwald H, Pearson D, Beery WL, Cheadle A. Youth development, community engagement, and reducing risk behavior. *J Prim Prev.* 2006;27:3–25

3. Gallagher K, Stanley A, Shearer D, Mosca C. Implementation of youth development programs: promise and challenges. *J Adolesc Health.* 2005;37(3 suppl):S61–S68
4. Johnston-Nicholson H, Collins C, Holmer H. Youth as people: the protective aspects of youth development in after-school programming. *Ann Am Acad Pol Soc Sci.* 2004;(591):55–71
5. Checkoway B. Youth participation as social justice. *Community Youth Dev J.* 2005:15–17
6. Fund for the City of New York. *A Guided Tour of Youth Development.* 2nd ed. New York, NY: Youth Development Institute; 1998
7. Hamilton S. Youth development and prevention. *J Public Health Manag Pract.* 2006;(suppl): S7–S9
8. Roth JL, Brooks-Gunn J. Youth development programs: risk, prevention and policy. *J Adolesc Health.* 2003;32:170–182
9. Search Institute. Forty developmental assets. Available at: www.search-institute.org/assets/forty.html. Accessed December 4, 2006
10. Connell J, Gambone M. Youth development in community settings: a community action framework. Available at: www.ydsi.org/YDSI/pdf/publication_02.pdf. Accessed February 1, 2007
11. Bernat DH, Resnick MD. Healthy youth development: science and strategies. *J Public Health Manag Pract.* 2006;(suppl):S10–S16
12. Lenhart A, Madden M, Hitlin P. Pew Internet & American Life Project: teens and technology— youth are leading the transition to a fully wired and mobile nation. Available at: www.pewinternet.org/pdfs/PIP_Teens_Tech_July2005web.pdf. Accessed May 29, 2007
13. Borzekowski DL, Rickert VI. Urban girls, Internet use and accessing health information. *J Pediatr Adolesc Gynecol.* 2000;13:94–95
14. Borzekowski DL, Rickert VI. Adolescent cybersurfing for health information: a new resource that crosses barriers. *Arch Pediatr Adolesc Med.* 2001;155:813–817
15. Bleakley A, Merzel CR, VanDevanter NL, Messeri P. Computer access and Internet use among urban youths. *Am J Public Health.* 2004;94:744–746
16. Skinner H, Biscope S, Poland B, Goldberg E. How adolescents use technology for health information: implications for health professionals from focus group studies. *J Med Internet Res.* 2003;5:e32. Available at: www.jmir.org/2003/4/e32
17. YMCA of the USA. Youth and technology. Available at: www.ymca.net/downloads/technology_strategy_paper.pdf. Accessed December 4, 2006
18. Valaitis R. Computers and the Internet: tools for youth empowerment. *J Med Internet Res.* 2005;7:e51. Available at: www.jmir.org/2005/5/e51
19. Becker HJ. Who's wired and who's not: children's access to and use of computer technology. *Future Child.* 2000;10:44–75
20. Kaiser Family Foundation. Bridging the digital divide: new ConnectNet/Conectado campaign uses fun, engaging tools to connect teens with computers and Internet [press release]. Available at: http://kff.org/entpartnerships/upload/Bridging-the-Digital-Divide-New-ConnectNet-Conectado-Campaign-Uses-Fun-Engaging-Tools-to-Connect-Teens-With-Computers-and-Internet.pdf. Accessed May 29, 2007
21. National Telecommunications and Information Administration. *A Nation Online: Entering the Broadband Age.* Washington, DC: National Telecommunications and Information Administration; 2004. Available at: www.ntia.doc.gov/reports/anol/NationOnlineBroadband04.pdf. Accessed February 1, 2007
22. Hall G. Teens and technology: preparing for the future. *New Dir Youth Dev.* 2006;(111):41–52, 8
23. McCord C, Freeman HP. Excess mortality in Harlem. *N Engl J Med.* 1990;322:173–177
24. Blum RW, Beuhring T, Shew MC, et al. The effects of race/ethnicity, income, and family structure on adolescent risk behaviors. *Am J Public Health.* 2000;90:1879–1884
25. Resnick MD, Bearman PS, Blum RW, et al. Protecting adolescents from harm: findings from the National Longitudinal Study on Adolescent Health. *JAMA.* 1997;278:823–832

A

B

C